PALEO AUTOIMMUNE PROTOCOL DIET

BY KEVIN WAGONFOOT

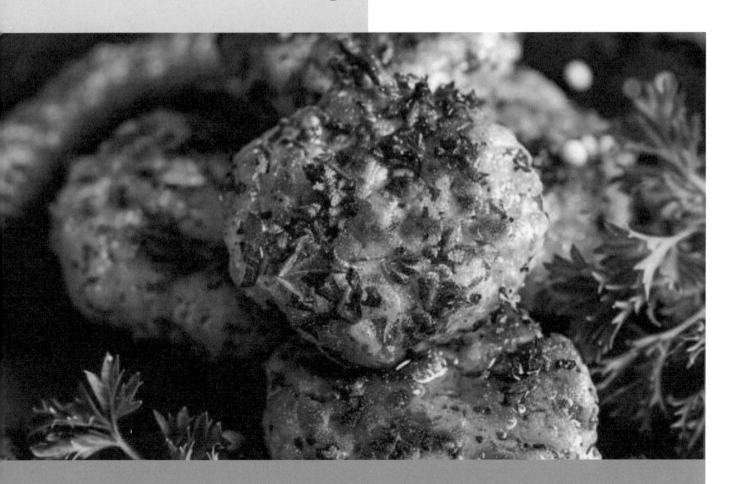

WELCOME

In my early twenties, I faced significant health challenges. I was overweight, constantly battling inflammation, and experiencing chronic fatigue. These issues often left me feeling frustrated and defeated. It was a difficult period in my life, but it also marked the beginning of a transformative journey.

Determined to reclaim my health, I decided to explore how diet could impact my well-being. I immersed myself in extensive research and experimented with various dietary approaches. This quest for knowledge and a better quality of life led me to discover the transformative power of specialized nutrition plans tailored to individual needs.

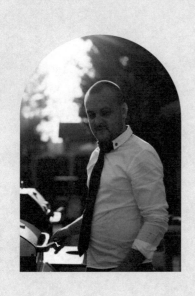

ABOUT ME

I believe food is more than fuel; it's key to optimal health and happiness. Everyone deserves to feel their best, starting with their diet. My approach emphasizes balanced, sustainable eating with whole foods, mindful eating, and the joy of cooking.

Kevin Wagonfoot

My life changed when I stumbled upon the Paleo Autoimmune Protocol (AIP) diet. The principles of AIP resonated with me, offering a comprehensive approach to managing autoimmune conditions through diet. By eliminating certain foods and focusing on nutrient-dense, anti-inflammatory options, AIP provided a structured path to healing.

Through my journey, I learned that the right diet can have a profound impact on health. I experienced firsthand the benefits of tailored nutrition plans. My inflammation reduced, my energy levels increased, and I began to feel like myself again. This personal transformation fueled my passion to help others achieve similar results.

I decided to write this book to share my insights and experiences with a wider audience. I want to provide a practical guide for those struggling with autoimmune conditions, offering them the tools and knowledge to improve their health through diet.

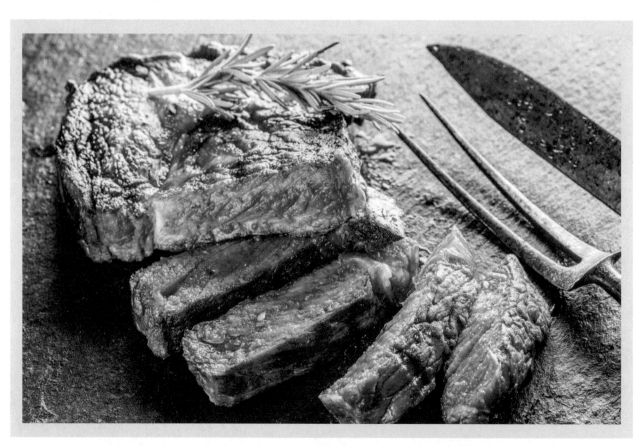

As a special bonus I have created an email series with an **additional two weeks of Paleo friendly recipes**. Each week you will receive a shopping list and meal plan for the week and then each day you'll get easy to follow and prepare recipes for that day in your inbox! Sign up right now, or wait until you have cooked your way through this book.

And to make the offer even sweeter I will be giving everyone on my mailing list updates and discounts on all my new healthy cookbooks as they are released!

Scan the code below to Sign Up now

Kevin Wagonfoot

TABLE OF CONTENTS

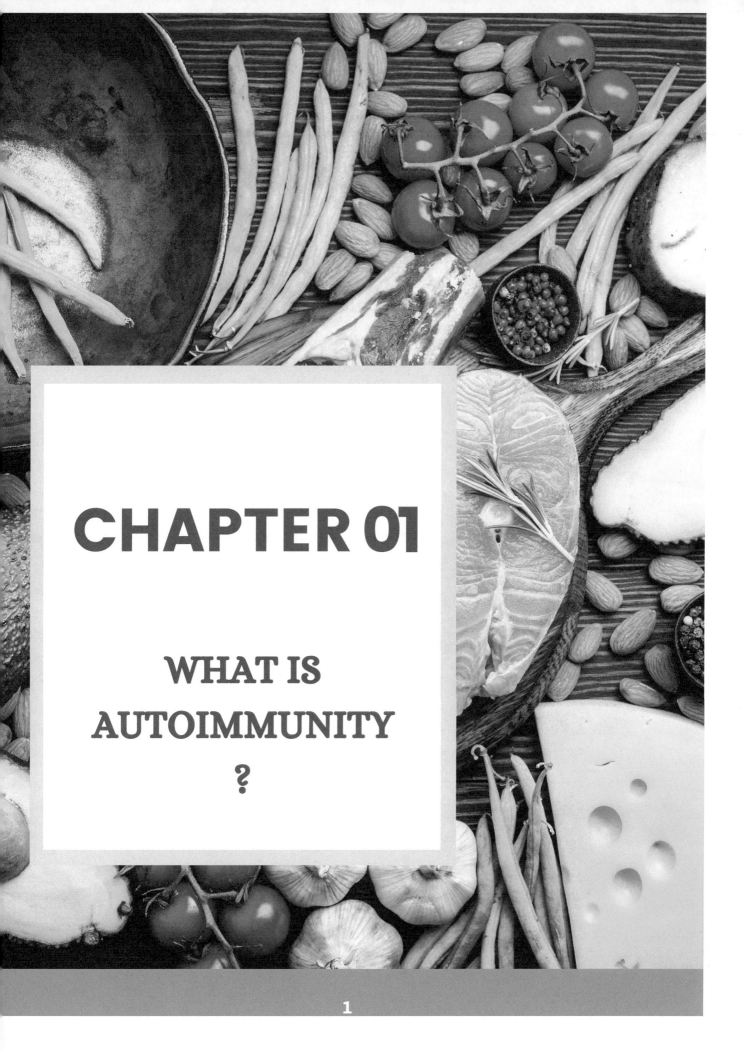

CHAPTER 01

WHAT IS AUTOIMMUNITY ?

UNDERSTANDING YOUR IMMUNE SYSTEM

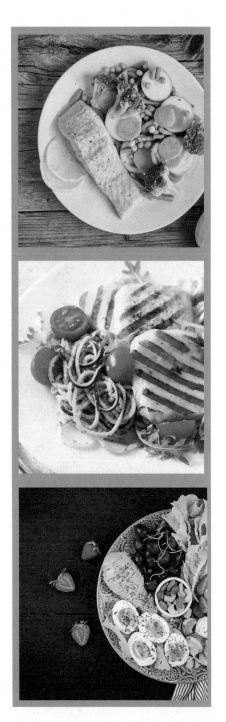

Autoimmunity is when the immune system mistakenly attacks the body's own tissues. Normally, it protects us from harmful invaders like bacteria and viruses by identifying and destroying them. In autoimmune conditions, it gets confused and attacks healthy cells instead.

To understand autoimmunity, it's important to know about the immune system. The immune system uses cells and proteins to protect the body by attacking harmful invaders. This process involves inflammation, which helps fight infections and heal injuries, causing redness, swelling, and pain.

In autoimmune diseases, this process goes wrong. The immune system starts targeting the body's own cells, leading to chronic inflammation and damage to healthy tissues. This can happen in any part of the body, depending on the specific autoimmune disease. For example, in rheumatoid arthritis, the immune system attacks the joints, causing pain and swelling. In type 1 diabetes, it attacks the insulin-producing cells in the pancreas.

COMMON AI DISEASES

Rheumatoid arthritis

This condition affects the joints, causing pain, stiffness, and swelling. Over time, it can lead to joint damage.

Lupus

Can affect various parts of the body, including the skin, joints, kidneys, and other organs. Symptoms can vary widely but often include fatigue, joint pain, and skin rashes.

Multiple sclerosis (MS)

The immune system attacks the protective covering of nerve fibers in the brain and spinal cord. This can lead to problems with movement, coordination, and vision.

Type 1 diabetes

Occurs when the immune system attacks the insulin-producing cells in the pancreas, leading to high blood sugar levels. People with type 1 diabetes need to take insulin to manage their blood sugar.

Hashimoto's thyroiditis

This condition affects the thyroid gland, leading to an underactive thyroid (hypothyroidism). Symptoms can include fatigue, weight gain, and depression.

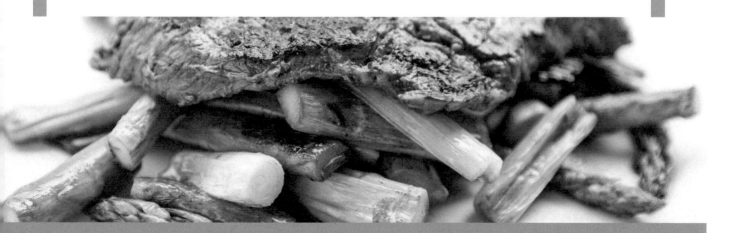

PRINCIPLES OF AIP

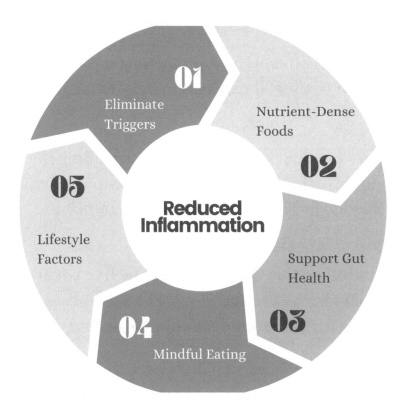

01 Eliminate Triggers

02 Nutrient-Dense Foods

03 Support Gut Health

04 Mindful Eating

05 Lifestyle Factors

Reduced Inflammation

ELIMINATION OF POTENTIAL TRIGGERS

The AIP diet removes foods that are known to cause inflammation or trigger immune responses. This includes:

- **Grains** (such as wheat, rice, and corn)
- **Legumes** (such as beans, lentils, and peanuts)
- **Dairy** products
- **Nuts** and **seeds**
- **Nightshades** (such as tomatoes, potatoes, eggplants, and peppers)
- **Eggs**
- **Processed foods** and food additives

FOCUS ON NUTRIENT-DENSE FOODS

The AIP diet emphasizes foods that are rich in vitamins, minerals, and other essential nutrients. These foods help support the immune system and overall health. Key nutrient-dense foods include:

- A wide variety of **vegetables** (excluding nightshades)
- High-quality **meats** and **seafood** (preferably grass-fed, pasture-raised, and wild-caught)
- **Organ meats** (such as liver and heart)
- **Fermented foods** (such as sauerkraut and kimchi)
- Healthy fats (such as olive oil, coconut oil, and avocado oil)

MINDFUL EATING

The AIP diet encourages mindful eating practices, such as taking the time to prepare your own meals, eating slowly, and paying attention to how different foods make you feel. This can help you develop a healthier relationship with food and become more attuned to your body's needs.

SUPPORTING GUT HEALTH

Crucial for overall health, especially for people with autoimmune conditions. The AIP diet aims to support gut health by eliminating foods that can irritate the gut lining and including foods that promote a healthy gut microbiome. This includes:

- **Bone broth**, which is rich in nutrients that support gut healing
- **Fermented foods**, which provide beneficial bacteria to support a healthy gut microbiome
- Plenty of **fiber-rich vegetables**, which help feed the beneficial bacteria in the gut

LIFESTYLE FACTORS

In addition to dietary changes, the AIP diet also emphasizes the importance of other lifestyle factors that can affect autoimmune health:

- Getting enough **sleep**
- Managing **stress**
- Regular **physical activity**
- Practicing **mindfulness and relaxation techniques**

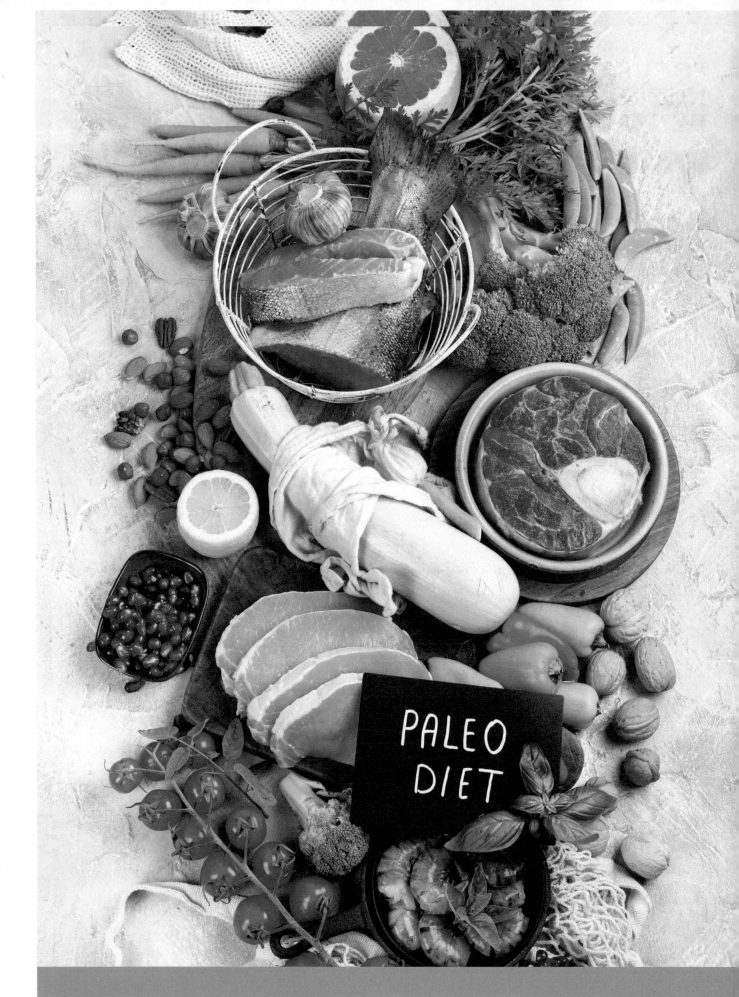

TRACK FOOD REACTIONS

Tracking and interpreting food reactions is an essential part of managing autoimmune conditions, especially when following the Paleo Autoimmune Protocol (AIP) diet. By monitoring how your body responds to different foods, you can identify which foods are beneficial and which ones may trigger symptoms. Here's how to effectively track and interpret your food reactions.

Autoimmune conditions can make your body sensitive to certain foods, which can cause inflammation and worsen symptoms. By tracking your food reactions, you can:

- **Identify foods that trigger symptoms**
- **Understand how different foods affect your body**
- **Make informed dietary choices**
- **Improve your overall health and well-being**

To track your food reactions, you'll need to keep a detailed food diary. Here's how to get started:

Keep a Food Diary
A food diary is a daily record of everything you eat and drink, along with any symptoms you experience. You can use a notebook, a spreadsheet, or a smartphone app to keep track.

Be Consistent
Consistency is key when tracking food reactions. Record everything you eat and drink every day, even if you think a food is harmless. This will help you identify patterns and make connections between foods and symptoms.

Identify Patterns
After a few weeks of tracking, review your food diary to identify patterns. Look for correlations between what you eat and how you feel. For example, if you notice that you experience joint pain after eating certain foods, those foods might be triggering your symptoms.

All recipes in this book include notes on any ingredients that might be reintroduced. If you are in the elimination phase of the AIP diet, you can omit these ingredients or choose another recipe.

When you begin the reintroduction phase, be sure to note how you react to these ingredients as they are reintroduced.

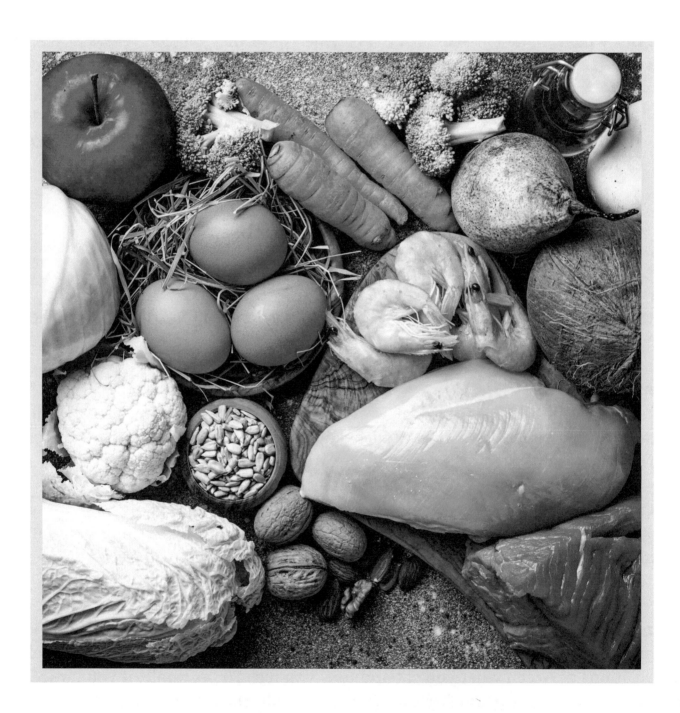

ASSESSMENT

Monitor for any digestive issues such as bloating, gas, diarrhea, constipation, or stomach pain. These can be signs of food intolerance.

1   2   3   4   5

Observe your skin for any changes such as rashes, acne, itching, or hives. Skin reactions can indicate an immune response.

1   2   3   4   5

Take note of any new or worsening joint or muscle pain. Increased inflammation in these areas can signal a problem with the reintroduced food.

1   2   3   4   5

Track any changes in your energy levels. Feeling unusually fatigued or experiencing a significant energy crash can be a reaction to a food.

1   2   3   4   5

Pay attention to mood swings, anxiety, depression, or brain fog. Mental and emotional changes can be linked to food sensitivities.

1   2   3   4   5

Assess any disruptions in your sleep patterns. Difficulty falling asleep, staying asleep, or experiencing restless sleep can be a sign of food intolerance.

1   2   3   4   5

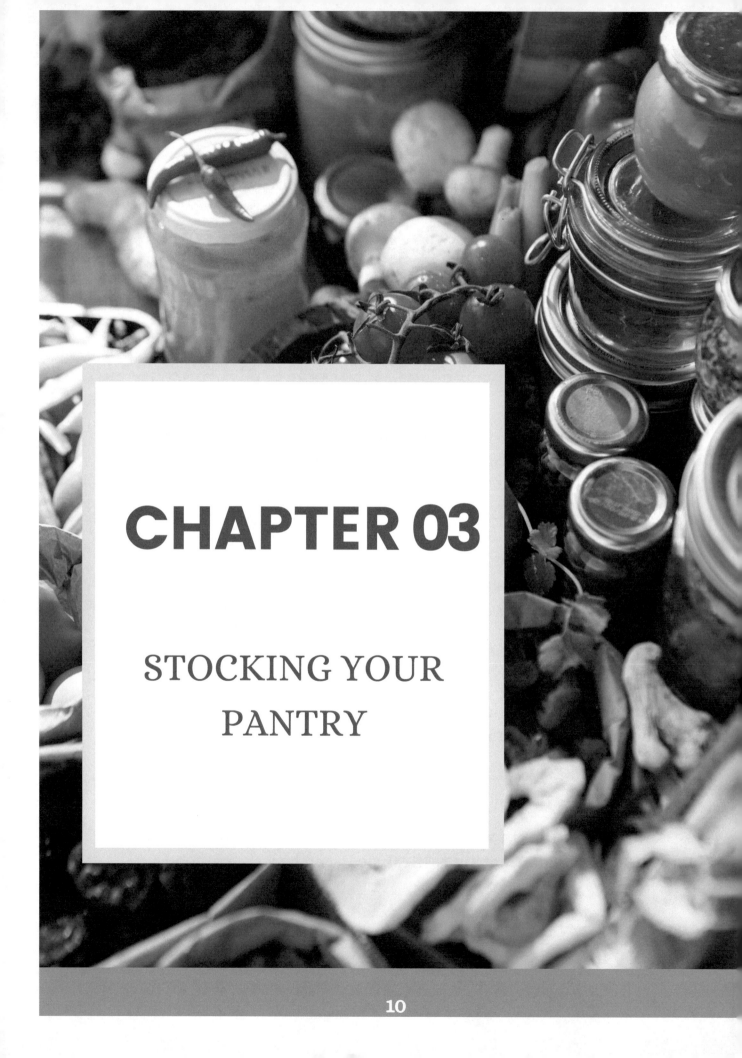

CHAPTER 03

STOCKING YOUR PANTRY

STOCKING YOUR PANTRY

HEALTHY FATS

- Extra virgin olive oil
- Coconut oil
- Avocado oil
- Lard or tallow from pastured animals

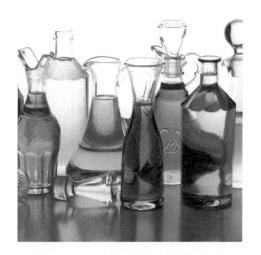

AIP-FRIENDLY FLOURS AND THICKENERS

- Coconut flour
- Cassava flour
- Tigernut flour
- Arrowroot powder
- Tapioca starch

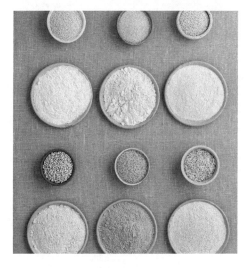

NATURAL SWEETENERS

- Honey (in moderation)
- Maple syrup (in moderation)
- Coconut sugar (in moderation)

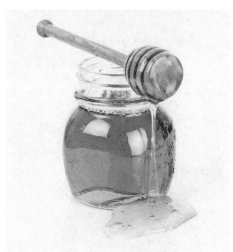

HERBS AND SPICES

- Basil
- Oregano
- Thyme
- Rosemary
- Sage
- Parsley
- Cilantro
- Cloves
- Dill (leaves, not seeds)
- Garlic powder (not garlic salt)
- Onion powder
- Ginger
- Turmeric
- Cinnamon

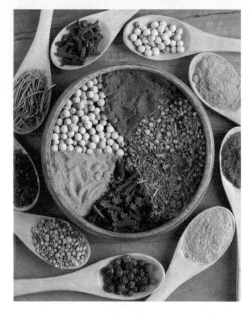

PANTRY STAPLES

- Canned coconut milk (ensure it's free from additives)
- Canned fish (like tuna or salmon, in water or olive oil)
- Applesauce (unsweetened)
- Coconut aminos (a soy sauce alternative)
- Bonebroth
- Baking soda
- Cream of tartar

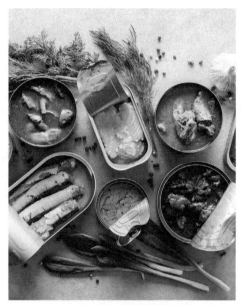

BEVERAGES

- Herbal teas (peppermint, chamomile, ginger)
- Green tea (in moderation)
- Coconut water

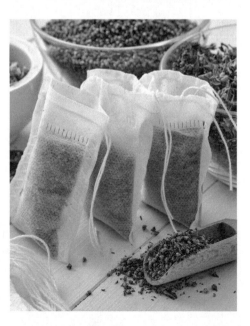

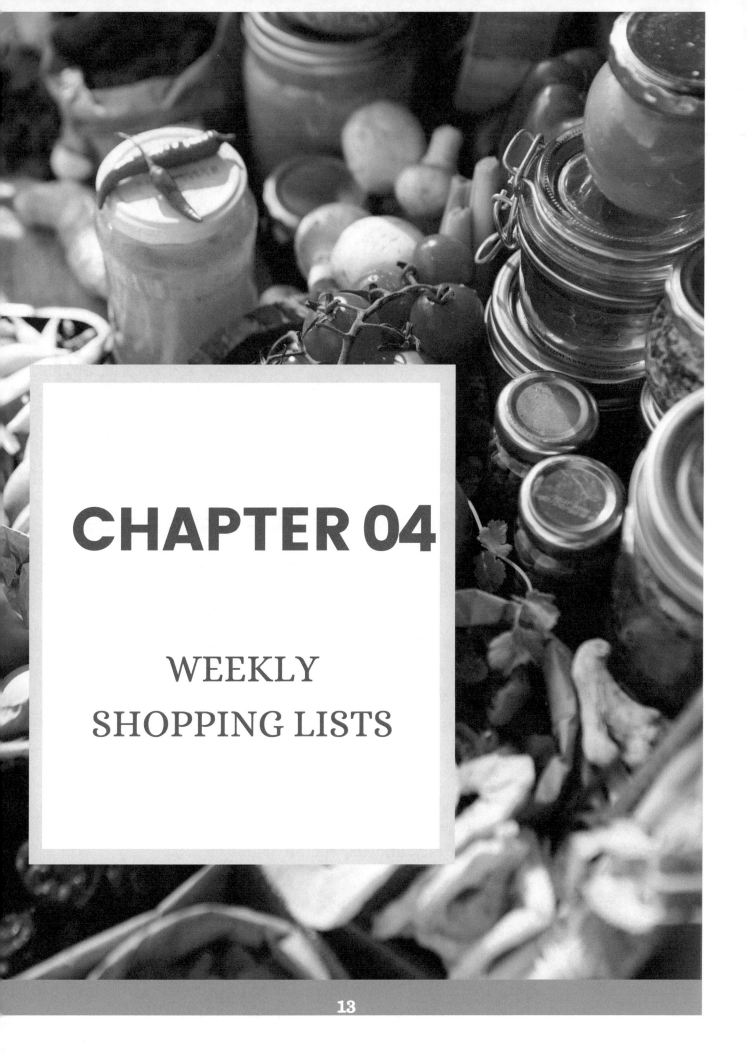

CHAPTER 04

WEEKLY
SHOPPING LISTS

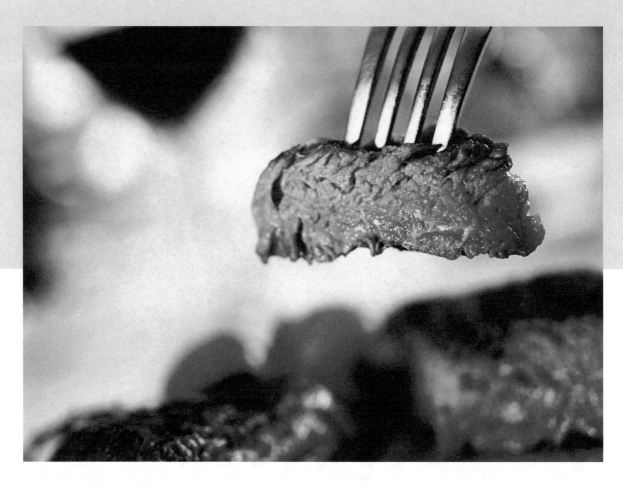

Welcome to the shopping list and meal planning chapter! Here's how you can use this book to make your weekly meal planning easy and stress-free.

Each week, you'll find a shopping list that includes all the ingredients you'll need for the recipes. Following the shopping list, there's a breakdown of daily meals for the week, organized on a 7-day calendar. Each meal will have a reference page number for the recipe, making it easy to find and prepare.

All recipes in this book include notes on any ingredients that might be reintroduced. If you are in the elimination phase of the AIP diet, you can skip these ingredients or pick another recipe.

When you start the reintroduction phase, be sure to note how you react to the ingredients as you add them back into your diet. This will help you understand what works best for your body. Happy cooking and planning!

WEEK ONE SHOPPING LIST

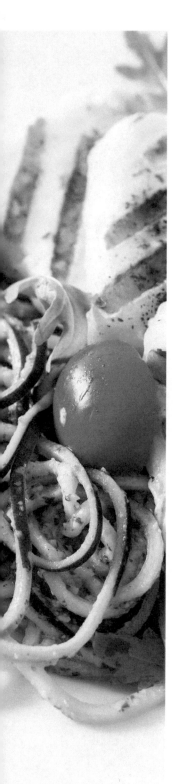

Proteins

- Salmon fillets: 3
- Salmon (canned): 1 can
- Ground chicken: 1 1/2 lbs
- Chicken breasts: 4
- Chicken thighs: 4

Vegetables

- Sweet potatoes: 6
- Garlic cloves: 22
- Broccoli heads: 2
- Cauliflower heads: 2
- Green onions: 2 bunches
- Brussels sprouts: 2 lbs
- Carrots: 8
- Celery stalks: 5
- Asparagus: 2 lbs
- Bell peppers: 2
- Zucchini: 4
- Leeks: 2
- Cabbage heads: 1
- Cucumbers: 5
- Beets: 3
- Spinach: 1 bunch
- Lettuce heads: 1
- Kale: 1 bunch

Fruits

- Avocados: 5
- Apples: 4
- Lemons: 11
- Blueberries: 1 pint
- Strawberries: 1 pint
- Bananas: 5
- Pears: 2
- Pineapple: 1
- Orange: 1

Herbs and Spices

- Fresh thyme: 1 bunch
- Fresh rosemary: 1 bunch
- Fresh basil: 1 bunch
- Fresh parsley: 1 bunch
- Fresh cilantro: 1 bunch
- Fresh dill: 1 bunch
- Fresh mint: 1 bunch
- Fresh ginger: 1 piece
- Cinnamon: 1 tsp
- Garlic powder: 1 tsp

Other

- Coconut yogurt: 1 cup
- Coconut water: 2 cups

WEEK ONE MEAL PLAN

	BREAKFAST	LUNCH	DINNER	SNACK
DAY 1	Sweet Potato and Apple Hash page 24	Chicken Salad with Avocado and Fresh Herbs page 53	Baked Salmon with Garlic and Herb Sweet Potatoes page 82	Carrot and Cucumber Sticks with Avocado Dip page 111
DAY 2	Green Smoothie with Spinach and Avocado page 25	Cauliflower Rice Bowl with Salmon and Vegetables page 54	Chicken Stir-Fry with Broccoli and Cauliflower page 83	Roasted Sweet Potato Chips page 113
DAY 3	Breakfast Sausage Patties with Sautéed Kale page 26	Chicken and Vegetable Soup page 55	Garlic and Herb Roasted Chicken with Brussels Sprouts page 84	Sautéed Kale Chips with Sea Salt page 114
DAY 4	Zucchini and Carrot Fritters page 27	Sweet Potato and Brussels Sprout Salad page 56	Grilled Lemon Herb Chicken with Asparagus page 85	Pear Slices with Fresh Cilantro page 115
DAY 5	Garlic and Herb Roasted Asparagus with Avocado page 28	Roasted Beet and Carrot Salad with Fresh Parsley page 59	Cauliflower Rice Stuffed Peppers page 86	Baked Apple Chips with Cinnamon page 116
DAY 6	Beet and Carrot Smoothie page 29	Broccoli and Apple Salad with Coconut Aminos Dressing page 57	Baked Chicken with Lemon and Fresh Thyme page 87	Cucumber Slices with Fresh Dill page 117
DAY 7	Banana and Blueberry Muffins page 30	Grilled Chicken and Asparagus Salad page 58	Roasted Garlic Chicken with Cabbage and Carrots page 88	Banana with Coconut Yogurt page 112

WEEK TWO SHOPPING LIST

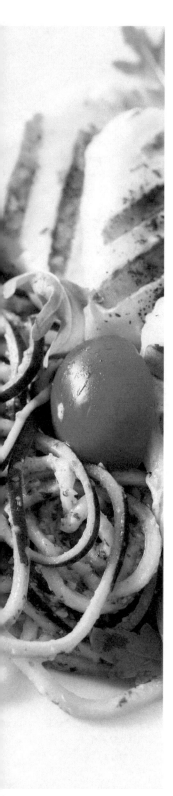

Proteins
- 2lb ground turkey
- 2lb turkey breast
- 2 cod fillets

Vegetables
- 6 sweet potatoes
- 2 zucchinis
- 2 bell peppers
- 1 small cabbage (green)
- 1 butternut squash
- 1 bunch asparagus
- 1 head broccoli
- 1 head cauliflower
- 1 bunch green onions
- 2 cups Brussels sprouts
- 2 cups spinach
- 4 cups kale
- 2 cups chard
- 2 carrots
- 2 celery stalks
- 1 cucumber
- 1 lemon
- 1 lime
- 2 beets
- 1 red onion
- 2 cloves garlic

Fruits
- Avocados: 5
- 4 apples
- 2 bananas
- 2 box strawberries
- 1 box blueberries
- 1 box raspberries
- 2 oranges
- 1 pear
- 1 bag grapes

Herbs and Spices
- 1 bunch fresh thyme
- 1 bunch fresh basil
- 1 bunch fresh parsley
- 1 bunch fresh cilantro
- 1 bunch fresh mint
- 1 bunch fresh dill
- 1 bunch fresh rosemary

Other
- 1 can coconut milk
- 1 container coconut yogurt
- 1 container bone broth
- 1 jar honey
- 1 bottle balsamic vinegar (AIP compliant)

WEEK TWO
MEAL PLAN

	BREAKFAST	LUNCH	DINNER	SNACK
DAY 1	Turkey and Spinach Breakfast Hash P 31	Turkey and Kale Salad with Fresh Lemon Dressing p 60	Lemon Herb Cod with Garlic and Green Onions p 89	Fresh Pear Slices with Turkey Roll-Ups p 118
DAY 2	Sweet Potato and Avocado Breakfast Bowl p 32	Cod and Asparagus Grain-Free Tacos p 61	Turkey and Sweet Potato Shepherd's Pie p 90	Cucumber and Avocado Bites p 119
DAY 3	Strawberry Banana Smoothie p 33	Butternut Squash Soup p 62	Grilled Bell Peppers and Turkey Kebabs p 91	Blueberry and Coconut Energy Balls p 120
DAY 4	Blueberry and Chard Smoothie Bowl p 34	Cauliflower Rice and Veggie Stir-Fry with Fresh Basil p 63	Baked Cod with Fresh Dill and Zucchini Noodles p 92	Carrot and Celery Sticks with Fresh Parsley Dip p 121
DAY 5	Turkey and Zucchini Breakfast Patties p 35	Spinach and Strawberry Salad with Avocado p 64	Roasted Beets and Carrots with Fresh Thyme p 93	Orange and Fresh Mint Fruit Salad p 122
DAY 6	Broccoli and Cauliflower Breakfast Bake p 36	Brussels Sprouts and Turkey Skillet p 65	Turkey Stuffed Green Cabbage Rolls p 94	Fresh Grapes and Cashews p 123
DAY 7	Raspberries and Coconut Yogurt Parfait p 37	Green Cabbage and Apple Slaw with Fresh Mint p 66	Pineapple and Turkey Stir-Fry with Fresh Cilantro p 95	Apple Slices with Fresh Rosemary and Lemon Drizzle p 124

WEEK THREE SHOPPING LIST

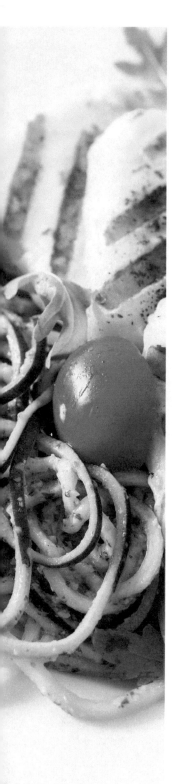

Proteins

- 2 lbs Chicken breasts
- 2 lbs Ground beef
- 1 lb Beef roast or steaks
- 4 Tilapia fillets
- 4 Eggs

Vegetables

- 1 head Broccoli
- 1 Cucumber
- 4 Sweet potatoes
- 4 Carrots
- 2 Celery stalks
- 2 Zucchini
- 3 cups Spinach
- 1 head Green cabbage
- 1 Butternut squash
- 6 Asparagus spears

Fruits

- 1 Mango
- 2 cups Pineapple
- 2 cups Strawberries
- 3 Avocados
- 3 Apples
- 2 Oranges
- 2 Limes
- 2 Lemons
- 3 Avocado

Herbs and Spices

- 1 tbsp Fresh dill
- 2 tbsp Fresh thyme
- 3 tbsp Fresh basil
- 1 tbsp Fresh rosemary
- 2 tbsp Fresh parsley
- 2 tbsp Fresh cilantro
- 5 Garlic cloves

Other

- Bone broth
- White rice
- Coconut milk
- Almond milk

WEEK THREE MEAL PLAN

	BREAKFAST	LUNCH	DINNER	SNACK
DAY 1	Beef and Asparagus Frittata P 38	Tilapia and Cucumber Wraps p 67	Stuffed Cabbage Rolls with Beef p 96	Pineapple and Strawberry Fruit Salad p 125
DAY 2	Sweet Potato and Apple Breakfast Bake p 39	Sweet Potato and Carrot Soup p 68	Beef and Green Cabbage Stir-Fry p 97	Cucumber and Avocado Slices with Fresh Dill p 126
DAY 3	Mango and Pineapple Parfait p 40	Avocado and Chicken Salad p 69	Sweet Potato and Beef Casserole p 98	Carrot and Celery Sticks with Guacamole p 127
DAY 4	Butternut Squash and Apple Porridge p 41	Zucchini Noodles with Fresh Basil and Beef p 70	Garlic and Herb Roasted Beef with Asparagus p 99	Blueberries and Fresh Thyme Compote p 128
DAY 5	Zucchini and Carrot Breakfast Muffins p 42	Green Bean and Beef Salad p 71	Butternut Squash and Beef Stew p 100	Bell Pepper Slices with Fresh Basil p 129
DAY 6	Strawberry and Lemon Chia Pudding p 43	Tilapia and Mango Salad p 72	Tomato and Beef Ragu p 101	Apple and Fresh Rosemary Infused Water p 130
DAY 7	Avocado and Beef Breakfast Wrap p 44	Broccoli and Beef Power Bowl p 73	Beef and Pineapple Skewers p 102	Orange and Lemon Zest Fruit Cups p 131

WEEK FOUR SHOPPING LIST

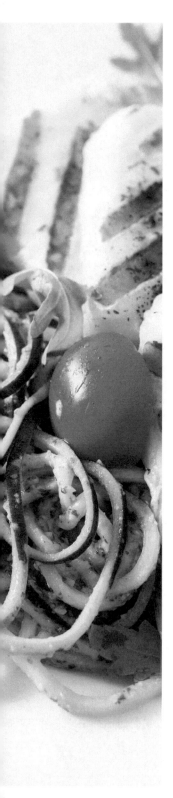

Proteins
- 2lb ground pork
- 1lb pork chops (boneless)
- 4 mahi-mahi fillets
- 4 eggs

Vegetables
- 4 sweet potatoes
- 3 onions
- 2 green onions
- 2 zucchini
- 2 bell peppers
- 2 cups spinach
- 3 carrots
- 2 beets
- 8 green cabbage leaves
- 1 cup cauliflower rice
- 1 cup broccoli
- 1 cup cherry tomatoes
- 1 cup green beans
- 1 bunch asparagus
- 2 cups butternut squash
- 2 cups Brussels sprouts
- 1 avocado
- 1 tomato
- 2 cups broccoli
- 2 cups cauliflower

Fruits
- 1 lemon (for juicing)
- 1 mango
- 1 bag grapes
- 2 kiwis
- 2 oranges
- 1 banana
- 1 box strawberries
- 1 box blueberries
- 1 pineapple
- 2 Apples

Herbs and Spices
- 1 package fresh parsley
- 1 package fresh rosemary
- 1 package fresh dill
- 1 package fresh thyme
- 1 package fresh cilantro
- 1 package fresh oregano
- 1 package fresh basil
- 1 package fresh mint

Other
- 1 cup bone broth
- 1 can chickpeas
- 1 package lentils
- 1 bag quinoa
- Quinoa bread
- Pine nuts (optional)
- Nutritional yeast
- Bag chia seeds (optional)

WEEK FOUR MEAL PLAN

	BREAKFAST	LUNCH	DINNER	SNACK
DAY 1	Broccoli and Cauliflower Scramble P 45	Sweet Potato and Brussels Sprouts Salad with Lemon Dressing p 74	Lemon Herb Mahi Mahi with Garlic and Green Onions p 103	Strawberry and Spinach Mini Skewers p 132
DAY 2	Sweet Potato and Carrot Pancakes p 46	Zucchini Noodles with Pesto and Cherry Tomatoes p 75	Pork and Sweet Potato Shepherd's Pie p 104	Zucchini Chips with Fresh Dill p 133
DAY 3	Strawberry and Banana Smoothie with Fresh Mint p 47	Broccoli and Cauliflower Soup with Fresh Thyme p 76	Grilled Bell Peppers and Pork Skewers p 105	Sweet Potato Fries with Fresh Thyme p 134
DAY 4	Zucchini and Apple Breakfast Muffins p 48	Beet and Orange Salad with Fresh Dill p 77	Baked Mahi Mahi with Fresh Dill and Zucchini Noodles p 106	Pineapple and Kiwi Fruit Salad p 135
DAY 5	Butternut Squash and Apple Porridge p 49	Pork and Asparagus Quinoa Bowl p 80	Roasted Beets and Carrots with Fresh Thyme p 107	Beet Chips with Fresh Oregano p 136
DAY 6	Avocado and Tomato Toast p 50	Butternut Squash and Lentil Stew p 78	Pork Stuffed Green Cabbage Rolls p 108	Mango and Grapes Fruit Salad p 137
DAY 7	Pineapple and Mango Smoothie Bowl p 51	Avocado and Green Bean Salad with Fresh Parsley p 79	Pineapple and Pork Stir-Fry with Fresh Cilantro p 109	Bell Pepper and Fresh Parsley Hummus Dip p 138

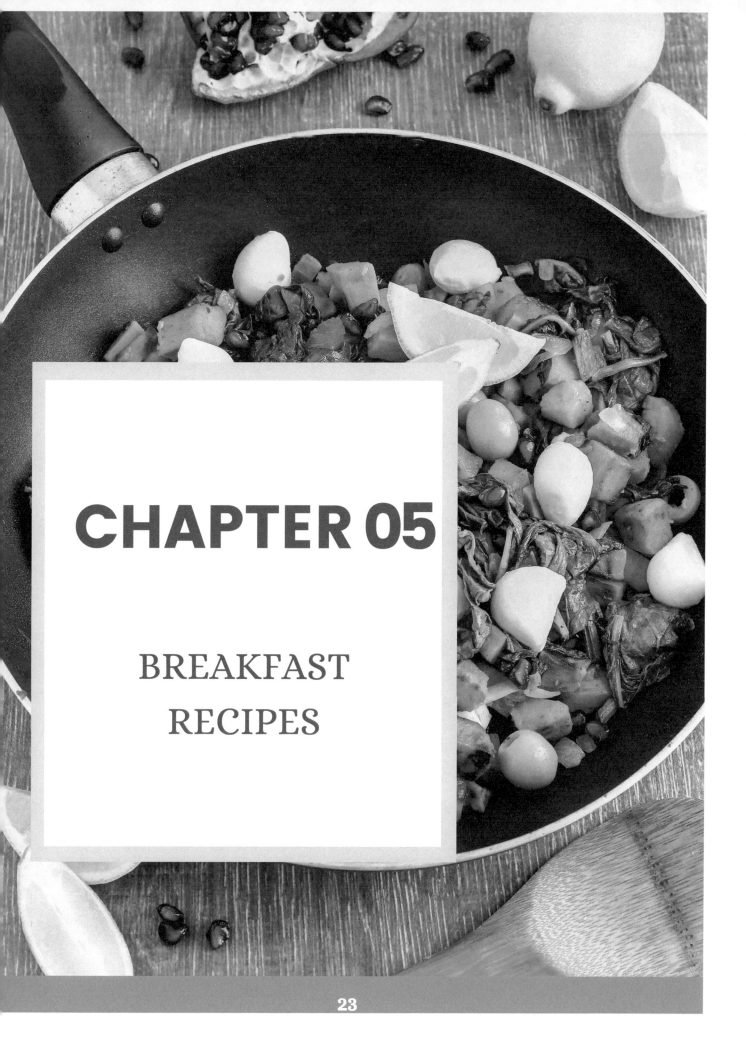

CHAPTER 05

BREAKFAST RECIPES

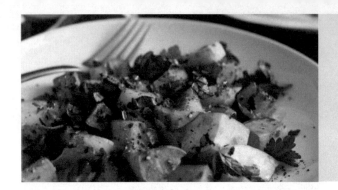

SWEET POTATO AND APPLE HASH

INGREDIENTS

COOK TIME: 15   TOTAL TIME: 25
PREP TIME: 10   SERVINGS: 2

- Sweet Potato (2 cups, diced)
- Apple (1, diced)
- Onion Powder (1 tsp)
- Coconut Oil (2 tbsp)
- Fresh Thyme (1 tsp)

DIRECTION

01   Heat coconut oil in a skillet over medium heat.

02   Add diced sweet potatoes and cook until slightly tender, about 10 minutes.

03   Add diced apple and onion powder.

04   Cook until apples are tender, about 5 minutes.

05   Stir in fresh thyme and serve hot.

NUTRITIONAL INFO PER SERVING

- Calories   250
- Protein   2g
- Carbs   45g
- Fat   10g
- Fiber   7g
- Sugar   10g

NOTES:
Store leftovers in an airtight container in the fridge for up to 2 days. Reheat in a skillet or microwave before serving.

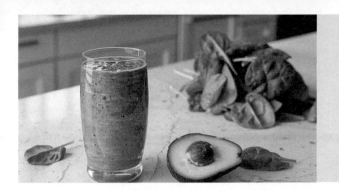

GREEN SMOOTHIE WITH SPINACH AND AVOCADO

INGREDIENTS

COOK TIME: 0
PREP TIME: 5
TOTAL TIME: 5
SERVINGS: 2

- Spinach (2 cups)

- Avocado (1)

- Coconut Water (1 cup)

- Lemon Juice (2 tbsp)

DIRECTION

01 Add spinach, avocado, coconut water, and lemon juice to a blender.

02 Blend until smooth and creamy.

03 Serve immediately.

NUTRITIONAL INFO PER SERVING

- Calories 200
- Protein 3g
- Carbs 20g
- Fat 12g
- Fiber 10g
- Sugar 5g

NOTES:

Best served fresh. Can be stored in the fridge for up to 24 hours, but separation may occur. Shake well before consuming.

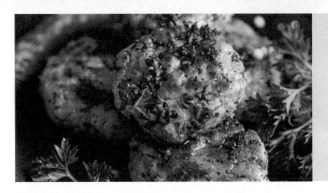

AIP BREAKFAST SAUSAGE PATTIES WITH SAUTÉED KALE

INGREDIENTS

COOK TIME: 20
PREP TIME: 10

TOTAL TIME: 30
SERVINGS: 2

- Ground Chicken (1 lb)
- Fresh Sage (1 tsp, chopped)
- Fresh Rosemary (1 tsp, chopped)
- Garlic Powder (1 tsp)
- Kale (2 cups, chopped)
- Coconut Oil (2 tbsp)

DIRECTION

01 Mix ground chicken with fresh sage, rosemary, and garlic powder in a bowl.

02 Form into small patties.

03 Heat coconut oil in a skillet over medium heat.

04 Cook patties for 5 minutes per side.

05 Remove patties and add kale to skillet.

06 Sauté kale until wilted, about 5 minutes.

NUTRITIONAL INFO PER SERVING

- Calories 350
- Protein 30g
- Carbs 10g
- Fat 20g
- Fiber 4g
- Sugar 1g

NOTES:

Store patties and kale separately in the fridge for up to 3 days. Reheat in a skillet or microwave before serving.

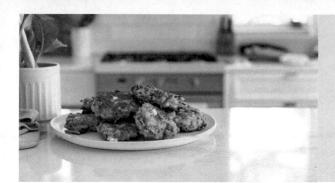

ZUCCHINI AND CARROT FRITTERS

INGREDIENTS

COOK TIME: 10
PREP TIME: 15
TOTAL TIME: 25
SERVINGS: 2

- Zucchini (2 cups, grated)
- Carrots (1 cup, grated)
- Coconut Flour (1/4 cup)
- Fresh Parsley (2 tbsp, chopped)
- Garlic Powder (1 tsp)
- Egg Replacer (1 tbsp + 3 tbsp water)
- Coconut Oil (2 tbsp)

DIRECTION

01 Mix grated zucchini and carrots with coconut flour, parsley, and garlic powder.

02 Prepare egg replacer according to package instructions.

03 Add egg replacer to veggie mix and combine.

04 Heat coconut oil in a skillet over medium heat.

05 Form mixture into small fritters.

06 Cook fritters for 3-4 minutes per side until golden.

NUTRITIONAL INFO PER SERVING

- Calories 180
- Protein 4g
- Carbs 20g
- Fat 9g
- Fiber 5g
- Sugar 4g

NOTES:

Store in an airtight container in the fridge for up to 3 days. Reheat in a skillet or oven before serving.

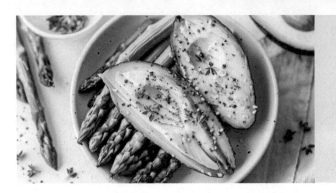

GARLIC AND HERB ROASTED ASPARAGUS WITH AVOCADO

INGREDIENTS

COOK TIME: 15 TOTAL TIME: 25
PREP TIME: 10 SERVINGS: 2

- Asparagus (1 bunch)
- Avocado (1)
- Garlic (2 cloves, minced)
- Fresh Rosemary (1 tsp, chopped)
- Fresh Thyme (1 tsp, chopped)
- Coconut Oil (2 tbsp)

DIRECTION

01 Preheat oven to 400°F (200°C).

02 Toss asparagus with coconut oil, garlic, rosemary, and thyme.

03 Spread on a baking sheet.

04 Roast for 15 minutes until tender.

05 Slice avocado and serve with roasted asparagus.

NUTRITIONAL INFO PER SERVING

- Calories   200
- Protein   3g
- Carbs   15g
- Fat   15g
- Fiber   8g
- Sugar   2g

NOTES:

Best served immediately. Store leftovers in the fridge for up to 2 days. Reheat in the oven before serving.

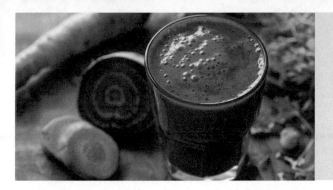

BEET AND CARROT SMOOTHIE

INGREDIENTS

COOK TIME: 0
PREP TIME: 5

TOTAL TIME: 5
SERVINGS: 2

- Beets (1 cup, cooked, diced)
- Carrots (1 cup, diced)
- Coconut Water (1 cup)
- Lemon Juice (2 tbsp)
- Fresh Ginger (1 tsp, grated)

DIRECTION

01 Add beets, carrots, coconut water, lemon juice, and fresh ginger to a blender.

02 Blend until smooth and creamy.

03 Serve immediately.

NUTRITIONAL INFO PER SERVING

- Calories   180
- Protein   3g
- Carbs   35g
- Fat   5g
- Fiber   7g
- Sugar   15g

NOTES:

Best served fresh. Can be stored in the fridge for up to 24 hours, but separation may occur. Shake well before consuming.

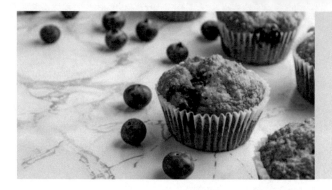

BANANA AND BLUEBERRY MUFFINS

INGREDIENTS

COOK TIME: 25   TOTAL TIME: 35
PREP TIME: 10   SERVINGS: 2

- Bananas (2, mashed)
- Blueberries (1 cup)
- Coconut Flour (1/2 cup)
- Baking Soda (1 tsp)
- Coconut Oil (1/4 cup)
- Lemon Juice (2 tbsp)
- Honey (2 tbsp)

DIRECTION

01   Preheat oven to 350°F (175°C).

02   Mix mashed bananas, coconut flour, baking soda, and coconut oil in a bowl.

03   Add lemon juice and honey, mix well.

04   Fold in blueberries.

05   Pour mixture into muffin tins.

06   Bake for 25 minutes or until golden.

NUTRITIONAL INFO PER SERVING

- Calories   220
- Protein   3g
- Carbs   35g
- Fat   10g
- Fiber   5g
- Sugar   15g

NOTES:

Store in an airtight container at room temperature for up to 3 days. Can be frozen for up to a month. Thaw before serving.

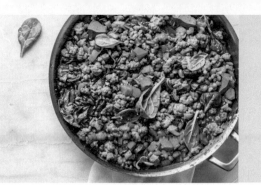

TURKEY AND SPINACH BREAKFAST HASH

INGREDIENTS

COOK TIME: 20
PREP TIME: 10
TOTAL TIME: 30
SERVINGS: 2

- 6 oz Ground turkey
- 2 cups Spinach (chopped)
- 1 Sweet potato (diced)
- 1/2 Onion (diced)
- 1 tbsp Olive oil
- 1/2 tsp Salt
- 1/4 tsp Black pepper (optional)

DIRECTION

01   Heat olive oil in a skillet over medium heat.

02   Add ground turkey and cook until browned.

03   Add sweet potato and onion; cook until tender.

04   Stir in spinach and cook until wilted.

05   Season with salt and black pepper (optional).

06   Serve hot.

NUTRITIONAL INFO PER SERVING

- Calories   350
- Protein   25g
- Carbs   30g
- Fat   15g
- Fiber   7g
- Sugar   4g

NOTES:
Store in an airtight container in the fridge for up to 3 days. Reheat in a skillet before serving.

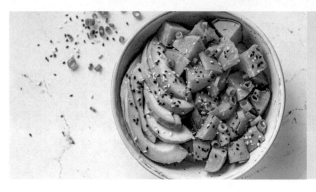

SWEET POTATO AND AVOCADO BREAKFAST BOWL

INGREDIENTS

COOK TIME: 20
PREP TIME: 10

TOTAL TIME: 30
SERVINGS: 2

- 2 Sweet potatoes (diced)
- 1 Avocado (sliced)
- 1 tbsp Olive oil
- 1/2 tsp Salt
- 1/4 tsp Garlic powder
- 1/4 tsp Paprika (if reintroduced)

DIRECTION

01   Preheat oven to 400°F (200°C).

02   Toss sweet potatoes with olive oil, salt, garlic powder, and paprika.

03   Bake for 20 minutes, until tender.

04   Divide roasted sweet potatoes into bowls.

05   Top with avocado slices.

06   Serve warm.

NUTRITIONAL INFO PER SERVING	
Calories	420
Protein	5g
Carbs	52g
Fat	22g
Fiber	10g
Sugar	7g

NOTES:

Store in an airtight container in the fridge for up to 2 days. Reheat in the oven or microwave before serving.

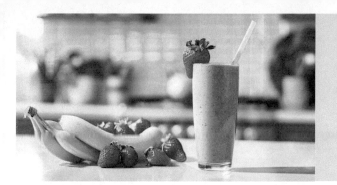

STRAWBERRY BANANA SMOOTHIE

INGREDIENTS

COOK TIME: 0
PREP TIME: 5

TOTAL TIME: 5
SERVINGS: 2

- 1 Banana
- 1 cup Strawberries (sliced)
- 1 cup Coconut milk
- 1 tbsp Honey

DIRECTION

01   Add all ingredients to a blender.

02   Blend until smooth.

03   Pour into glasses and serve.

NUTRITIONAL INFO PER SERVING

- Calories   220
- Protein   2g
- Carbs   45g
- Fat   5g
- Fiber   6g
- Sugar   28g

NOTES:

Best served immediately. Store any leftovers in the fridge for up to 1 day.

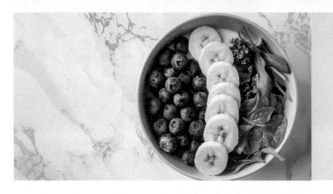

BLUEBERRY AND CHARD SMOOTHIE BOWL

INGREDIENTS

COOK TIME: 0   TOTAL TIME: 5
PREP TIME: 5   SERVINGS: 2

- 1 cup Blueberries
- 1 Banana
- 1 cup Chard (chopped)
- 1 cup Coconut milk
- 1 tbsp Honey
- 1 tsp Lemon juice

DIRECTION

01 Add blueberries, banana, chard, coconut milk, honey, and lemon juice to a blender.

02 Blend until smooth.

03 Pour into bowls and serve.

NUTRITIONAL INFO PER SERVING

- Calories 260
- Protein 3g
- Carbs 55g
- Fat 6g
- Fiber 8g
- Sugar 33g

NOTES:
Best served immediately. Store any leftovers in the fridge for up to 1 day.

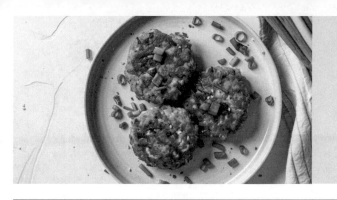

TURKEY AND ZUCCHINI BREAKFAST PATTIES

INGREDIENTS

COOK TIME: 15
PREP TIME: 10

TOTAL TIME: 25
SERVINGS: 2

- 6 oz Ground turkey
- 1 Zucchini (grated)
- 1/4 cup Green onions (chopped)
- 1/2 tsp Salt
- 1/4 tsp Black pepper (optional)
- 1 tbsp Olive oil

DIRECTION

01 Mix ground turkey, grated zucchini, green onions, salt, and black pepper (optional) in a bowl.

02 Form mixture into patties.

03 Heat olive oil in a skillet over medium heat.

04 Cook patties for 5-7 minutes on each side, until browned and cooked through.

05 Serve hot.

NUTRITIONAL INFO PER SERVING

- Calories 280
- Protein 20g
- Carbs 8g
- Fat 18g
- Fiber 2g
- Sugar 1g

NOTES:
Store patties in an airtight container in the fridge for up to 3 days. Reheat in a skillet before serving.

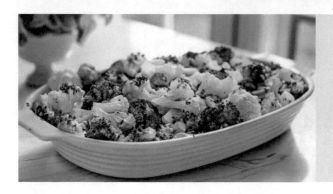

BROCCOLI AND CAULIFLOWER BREAKFAST BAKE

INGREDIENTS

COOK TIME: 30   TOTAL TIME: 40
PREP TIME: 10   SERVINGS: 2

- 1 cup Broccoli (chopped)
- 1 cup Cauliflower (chopped)
- 1/2 Onion (diced)
- 1 cup Coconut milk
- 1 tbsp Olive oil
- 1/2 tsp Salt
- 1/4 tsp Garlic powder
- 1/4 tsp Thyme

DIRECTION

01   Preheat oven to 375°F (190°C).

02   Heat olive oil in a skillet over medium heat.

03   Add broccoli, cauliflower, and onion; cook until tender.

04   Transfer to a baking dish.

05   Pour coconut milk over vegetables and season with salt, garlic powder, and thyme.

06   Bake for 30 minutes, until golden.

NUTRITIONAL INFO PER SERVING

- Calories   200
- Protein   4g
- Carbs   14g
- Fat   15g
- Fiber   5g
- Sugar   4g

NOTES:

Store in an airtight container in the fridge for up to 3 days. Reheat in the oven before serving.

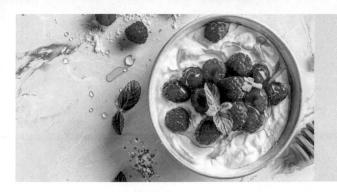

RASPBERRIES AND COCONUT YOGURT PARFAIT

INGREDIENTS

COOK TIME: 0
PREP TIME: 5
TOTAL TIME: 5
SERVINGS: 2

- 1 cup Raspberries
- 1 cup Coconut yogurt
- 1 tbsp Honey
- fresh mint sprig

DIRECTION

01 Layer raspberries and coconut yogurt in serving bowl.

02 Drizzle honey, place mint on top.

03 Serve immediately.

NUTRITIONAL INFO PER SERVING

- Calories 180
- Protein 2g
- Carbs 32g
- Fat 8g
- Fiber 6g
- Sugar 20g

NOTES:

Best served immediately. Store any leftover coconut yogurt in the fridge.

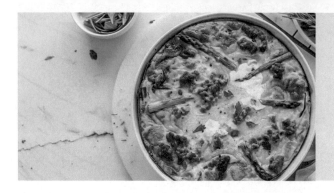

BEEF AND ASPARAGUS FRITTATA
(REINTRODUCTION: EGGS)

INGREDIENTS

COOK TIME: 15   TOTAL TIME: 25
PREP TIME: 10   SERVINGS: 2

- 4 oz Ground beef
- 6 Asparagus spears (chopped)
- 4 Eggs (beaten)
- 1/2 Onion (diced)
- 2 tbsp Olive oil
- 1/2 tsp Sea salt
- 1/4 tsp Black pepper (optional)
- 1 tbsp Fresh parsley (chopped)

DIRECTION

01 Preheat oven to 375°F (190°C).

02 Heat olive oil in a skillet over medium heat.

03 Add onion and asparagus; cook until tender.

04 Add ground beef and cook until browned.

05 Pour beaten eggs over the mixture.

06 Transfer skillet to oven and bake for 15 minutes.

NUTRITIONAL INFO PER SERVING

- Calories   350
- Protein   28g
- Carbs   10g
- Fat   26g
- Fiber   2g
- Sugar   2g

NOTES:

Store leftovers in an airtight container in the fridge for up to 2 days. Reheat in the oven before serving.

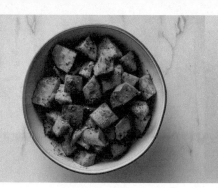

SWEET POTATO AND APPLE BREAKFAST BAKE

INGREDIENTS

COOK TIME: 30
PREP TIME: 10

TOTAL TIME: 40
SERVINGS: 2

- 2 Sweet potatoes (diced)
- 2 Apples (diced)
- 1 tbsp Coconut oil
- 1 tbsp Honey
- 1/2 tsp Cinnamon
- 1/4 tsp Nutmeg

DIRECTION

01   Preheat oven to 375°F (190°C).

02   Toss sweet potatoes and apples with coconut oil, honey, cinnamon, and nutmeg.

03   Spread mixture in a baking dish.

04   Bake for 30 minutes, until tender.

05   Serve warm.

NUTRITIONAL
INFO PER
SERVING

- Calories   250
- Protein   2g
- Carbs   52g
- Fat   6g
- Fiber   8g
- Sugar   22g

NOTES:
Store leftovers in an airtight container in the fridge for up to 2 days. Reheat in the oven before serving.

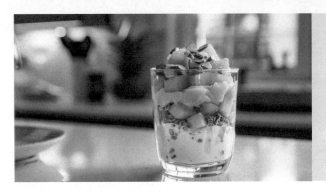

MANGO AND PINEAPPLE PARFAIT
(REINTRODUCTION: ALMOND MILK)

INGREDIENTS

COOK TIME: 0
PREP TIME: 10

TOTAL TIME: 10
SERVINGS: 2

- 1 Mango (diced)
- 1 cup Pineapple (diced)
- 1 cup Coconut yogurt
- 1/2 cup Almond milk
- 1 tbsp Honey
- 1/4 cup Almonds (chopped)

DIRECTION

01 In serving glasses, layer mango, pineapple, and coconut yogurt.

02 Drizzle with honey.

03 Top with chopped almonds.

04 Pour almond milk over parfait.

05 Serve immediately.

NUTRITIONAL INFO PER SERVING

- Calories   300
- Protein   5g
- Carbs   40g
- Fat   14g
- Fiber   6g
- Sugar   32g

NOTES:
Best served immediately. Store any leftover ingredients separately in the fridge.

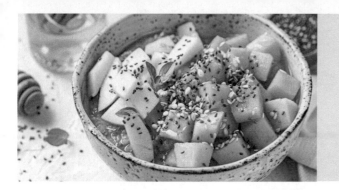

BUTTERNUT SQUASH AND APPLE PORRIDGE

(REINTRODUCTION: CHIA SEEDS)

INGREDIENTS

COOK TIME: 20
PREP TIME: 10
TOTAL TIME: 30
SERVINGS: 2

- 2 cups Butternut squash (diced)
- 2 Apples (diced)
- 2 tbsp Chia seeds
- 1 cup Coconut milk
- 1 tbsp Honey
- 1/2 tsp Cinnamon
- 1/4 tsp Nutmeg

DIRECTION

01 In a pot, combine butternut squash, apples, and coconut milk.

02 Bring to a boil, then simmer until squash is tender.

03 Stir in chia seeds, honey, cinnamon, and nutmeg.

04 Cook for 5 more minutes, stirring frequently.

05 Serve warm.

NUTRITIONAL INFO PER SERVING

- Calories 280
- Protein 4g
- Carbs 55g
- Fat 8g
- Fiber 10g
- Sugar 26g

NOTES:
Store in an airtight container in the fridge for up to 2 days. Reheat on the stovetop before serving.

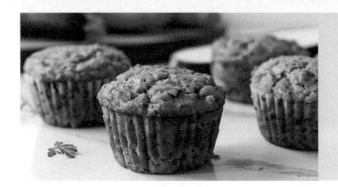

ZUCCHINI AND CARROT BREAKFAST MUFFINS
(EGG REINTRODUCTION)

INGREDIENTS

COOK TIME: 25   TOTAL TIME: 35
PREP TIME: 10   SERVINGS: 2

- 1 Zucchini (grated)
- 1 Carrot (grated)
- 2 Eggs (beaten)
- 1/2 cup Coconut flour
- 1 tbsp Honey
- 1/2 tsp Sea salt
- 1/4 tsp Baking soda
- 1/4 tsp Cinnamon

DIRECTION

01   Preheat oven to 350°F (175°C).

02   In a bowl, mix grated zucchini, carrot, beaten eggs, coconut flour, honey, sea salt, baking soda, and cinnamon.

03   Spoon batter into muffin tins.

04   Bake for 25 minutes or until a toothpick comes out clean.

05   Cool before serving.

NUTRITIONAL INFO PER SERVING

- Calories   220
- Protein   5g
- Carbs   25g
- Fat   10g
- Fiber   6g
- Sugar   8g

NOTES:
Store in an airtight container for up to 3 days. Reheat before serving.

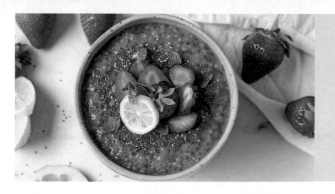

STRAWBERRY AND LEMON CHIA PUDDING

(REINTRODUCTION: CHIA SEEDS)

INGREDIENTS

COOK TIME: 0
PREP TIME: 10

TOTAL TIME: 10
SERVINGS: 2

- 1 cup Strawberries (sliced)
- 1 Lemon (juiced)
- 2 tbsp Chia seeds
- 1 cup Coconut milk
- 1 tbsp Honey

DIRECTION

01 In a bowl, mix coconut milk, lemon juice, chia seeds, and honey.

02 Stir in sliced strawberries.

03 Refrigerate for at least 2 hours or overnight.

04 Serve chilled.

NUTRITIONAL INFO PER SERVING

- Calories 200
- Protein 3g
- Carbs 20g
- Fat 10g
- Fiber 8g
- Sugar 14g

NOTES:
Store in an airtight container in the fridge for up to 2 days.

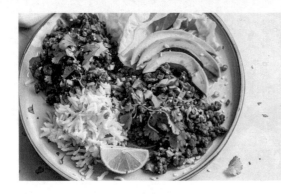

AVOCADO AND BEEF BREAKFAST WRAP

(REINTRODUCTION: WHITE RICE)

INGREDIENTS

COOK TIME: 10   TOTAL TIME: 20
PREP TIME: 10   SERVINGS: 2

- 4 oz Ground beef
- 1 Avocado (sliced)
- 1/2 cup White rice (cooked)
- 2 Lettuce leaves
- 1/2 tsp Sea salt
- 1/4 tsp Black pepper (optional)

- 1 tbsp Fresh cilantro (chopped)
- 1 Lime (quartered)

DIRECTION

01   Cook ground beef until browned, season with salt and pepper (optional).

02   Warm cooked white rice.

03   In a lettuce leaf, layer beef, avocado slices, and rice.

04   Sprinkle with fresh cilantro.

05   Serve with lime wedges.

NUTRITIONAL INFO PER SERVING

- Calories   350
- Protein   18g
- Carbs   32g
- Fat   18g
- Fiber   5g
- Sugar   2g

NOTES:
Store components separately in the fridge for up to 2 days. Assemble just before serving.

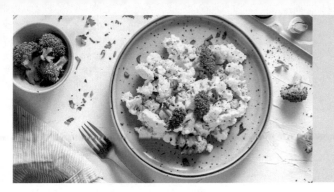

BROCCOLI AND CAULIFLOWER SCRAMBLE

(WITH EGGS – REINTRODUCTION)

INGREDIENTS

COOK TIME: 10
PREP TIME: 10
TOTAL TIME: 20
SERVINGS: 2

- 4 Eggs (beaten)
- 1 cup Broccoli (chopped)
- 1 cup Cauliflower (chopped)
- 1/2 Onion (diced)
- 2 tbsp Olive oil
- 1/2 tsp Sea salt
- 1/4 tsp Black pepper (optional)
- 1 tbsp Fresh parsley (chopped)

DIRECTION

01   Heat olive oil in a skillet over medium heat.

02   Add onion, broccoli, and cauliflower; cook until tender.

03   Pour beaten eggs over the vegetables.

04   Stir and cook until eggs are set.

05   Season with salt and pepper (optional).

06   Sprinkle with fresh parsley and serve.

NUTRITIONAL INFO PER SERVING

- Calories   300
- Protein   18g
- Carbs   12g
- Fat   22g
- Fiber   4g
- Sugar   3g

NOTES:
Store leftovers in an airtight container in the fridge for up to 2 days. Reheat in the skillet before serving.

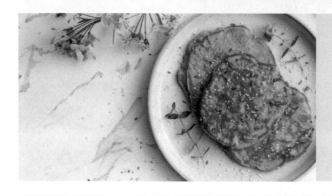

SWEET POTATO AND CARROT PANCAKES

INGREDIENTS

COOK TIME: 10
PREP TIME: 10
TOTAL TIME: 20
SERVINGS: 2

- 1 Sweet potato (grated)
- 1 Carrot (grated)
- 2 Eggs (beaten)
- 1/4 cup Coconut flour
- 1 tbsp Honey
- 1/2 tsp Cinnamon
- 1/4 tsp Nutmeg
- 1/4 tsp Sea salt
- 1 tbsp Coconut oil

DIRECTION

01 In a bowl, mix grated sweet potato, carrot, beaten eggs, coconut flour, honey, cinnamon, nutmeg, and sea salt.

02 Heat coconut oil in a skillet over medium heat.

03 Spoon batter into the skillet and cook pancakes until golden brown on both sides.

04 Serve warm.

NUTRITIONAL INFO PER SERVING

- Calories 250
- Protein 6g
- Carbs 36g
- Fat 10g
- Fiber 6g
- Sugar 10g

NOTES:
Store leftovers in an airtight container in the fridge for up to 2 days. Reheat in a skillet before serving.

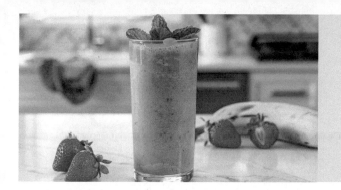

STRAWBERRY AND BANANA SMOOTHIE WITH FRESH MINT

INGREDIENTS

COOK TIME: 0   TOTAL TIME: 5
PREP TIME: 5   SERVINGS: 2

- 1 Banana
- 1 cup Strawberries (sliced)
- 1 cup Coconut milk
- 1 tbsp Fresh mint (chopped)
- 1 tbsp Honey

DIRECTION

01 Combine banana, strawberries, coconut milk, fresh mint, and honey in a blender.

02 Blend until smooth.

03 Pour into glasses and serve immediately.

NUTRITIONAL INFO PER SERVING

- Calories 200
- Protein 2g
- Carbs 36g
- Fat 6g
- Fiber 4g
- Sugar 22g

NOTES:

Best served immediately. Store leftovers in the fridge for up to 1 day.

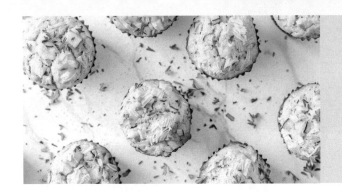

ZUCCHINI AND APPLE BREAKFAST MUFFINS

(WITH ALMOND MILK - REINTRODUCTION)

INGREDIENTS

COOK TIME: 25
PREP TIME: 10
TOTAL TIME: 35
SERVINGS: 2

- 1 Zucchini (grated)
- 1 Apple (grated)
- 2 Eggs (beaten)
- 1/2 cup Almond milk
- 1/2 cup Coconut flour
- 1 tbsp Honey
- 1/2 tsp Baking soda
- 1/2 tsp Cinnamon
- 1/4 tsp Sea salt

DIRECTION

01 Preheat oven to 350°F (175°C).

02 In a bowl, mix grated zucchini, apple, beaten eggs, almond milk, coconut flour, honey, baking soda, cinnamon, and sea salt.

03 Spoon batter into muffin tins.

04 Bake for 25 minutes or until a toothpick comes out clean.

05 Cool before serving.

NUTRITIONAL INFO PER SERVING

- Calories   220
- Protein   5g
- Carbs   28g
- Fat   10g
- Fiber   4g
- Sugar   12g

NOTES:
Store leftovers in an airtight container for up to 3 days. Reheat before serving.

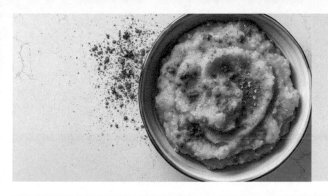

BUTTERNUT SQUASH AND APPLE POWER BOWL
(FOR REINTRODUCTION)

INGREDIENTS

COOK TIME: 20
PREP TIME: 10
TOTAL TIME: 30
SERVINGS: 2

- 2 cups Butternut squash (diced)
- 2 Apples (diced)
- 2 tbsp Chia seeds (optional)
- 1 cup Coconut milk
- 1 tbsp Honey
- 1/2 tsp Cinnamon
- 1/4 tsp Nutmeg
- 1/4 tsp Sea salt

DIRECTION

01 In a pot, combine butternut squash, apples, and coconut milk.

02 Bring to a boil, then simmer until squash is tender.

03 Stir in chia seeds (optional), honey, cinnamon, nutmeg, and sea salt.

04 Cook for 5 more minutes, stirring frequently.

05 Serve warm.

NUTRITIONAL INFO PER SERVING

- Calories 250
- Protein 4g
- Carbs 40g
- Fat 10g
- Fiber 8g
- Sugar 20g

NOTES:

Store in an airtight container in the fridge for up to 2 days. Reheat on the stovetop before serving.

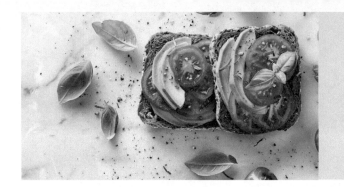

AVOCADO AND TOMATO TOAST
(WITH QUINOA BREAD – REINTRODUCTION)

INGREDIENTS

COOK TIME: 0
PREP TIME: 10
TOTAL TIME: 10
SERVINGS: 2

- 2 slices Quinoa bread
- 1 Avocado (sliced)
- 1 Tomato (sliced)
- 1 tbsp Lemon juice
- 1 tbsp Olive oil
- 1/4 tsp Sea salt
- 1/4 tsp Black pepper (optional)
- 1 tbsp Fresh basil (chopped)

DIRECTION

01 Toast quinoa bread slices.

02 In a bowl, toss avocado slices with lemon juice, olive oil, salt, and pepper (optional).

03 Layer avocado and tomato slices on toasted bread.

04 Sprinkle with fresh basil and serve.

NUTRITIONAL INFO PER SERVING

- Calories 300
- Protein 8g
- Carbs 34g
- Fat 18g
- Fiber 10g
- Sugar 4g

NOTES:
Best served immediately. Store leftover ingredients separately in the fridge for up to 1 day.

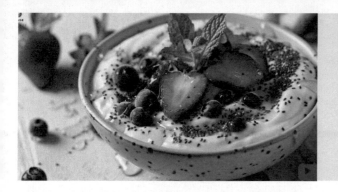

PINEAPPLE AND MANGO SMOOTHIE BOWL

(FOR REINTRODUCTION)

INGREDIENTS

COOK TIME: 0
PREP TIME: 10
TOTAL TIME: 10
SERVINGS: 2

- 1 cup Pineapple (diced)
- 1 cup Mango (diced)
- 1 cup Coconut milk
- 1 tbsp Honey
- 1/4 cup Blueberries
- 1/4 cup Strawberries (sliced)
- 1 tbsp Chia seeds (optional)
- 1 tbsp Fresh mint (chopped)

DIRECTION

01 Combine pineapple, mango, coconut milk, and honey in a blender.

02 Blend until smooth.

03 Pour into bowls and top with blueberries, strawberries, chia seeds (optional), and fresh mint.

04 Serve immediately.

NUTRITIONAL INFO PER SERVING

- Calories   300
- Protein   3g
- Carbs   50g
- Fat   10g
- Fiber   6g
- Sugar   35g

NOTES:

Best served immediately. Store leftovers in the fridge for up to 1 day.

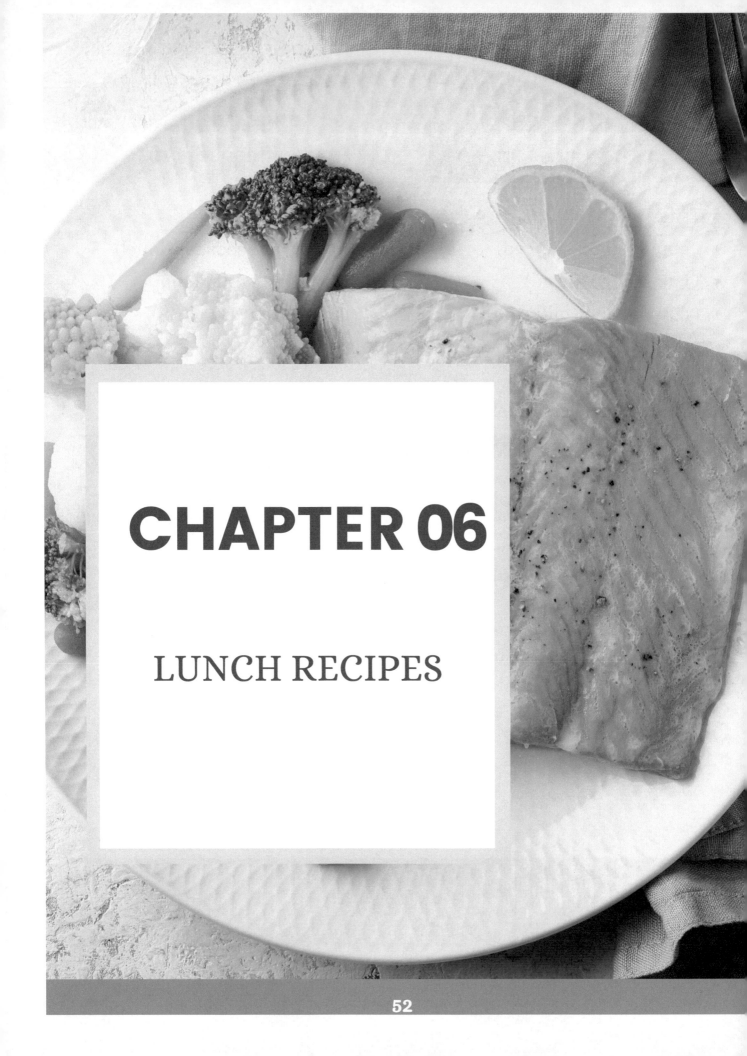

CHAPTER 06

LUNCH RECIPES

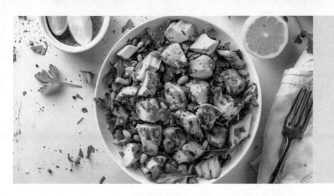

CHICKEN SALAD WITH AVOCADO AND FRESH HERBS

INGREDIENTS

COOK TIME: 0
PREP TIME: 10
TOTAL TIME: 10
SERVINGS: 2

- Chicken Breast (2, cooked, diced)
- Avocado (1, diced)
- Fresh Parsley (2 tbsp)
- Fresh Cilantro (2 tbsp)
- Lemon Juice (2 tbsp)
- Coconut Oil (2 tbsp)
- Salt (to taste)
- Pepper (to taste, optional)
- Pinenuts (reintroduction)

DIRECTION

01 In a large bowl, combine diced chicken, avocado, parsley, cilantro, and lemon juice.

02 Drizzle with coconut oil, add pine nuts (if using) and mix well.

03 Season with salt and pepper to taste.

04 Serve immediately.

NUTRITIONAL INFO PER SERVING

- Calories   350
- Protein   30g
- Carbs   10g
- Fat   20g
- Fiber   8g
- Sugar   2g

NOTES:
Best served fresh. Store leftovers in an airtight container in the fridge for up to 2 days.

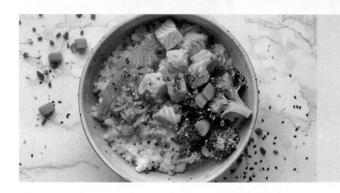

CAULIFLOWER RICE BOWL WITH SALMON AND VEGETABLES

INGREDIENTS

COOK TIME: 15   TOTAL TIME: 25
PREP TIME: 10   SERVINGS: 2

- Salmon (2 fillets)
- Cauliflower (2 cups, riced)
- Broccoli (1 cup, florets)
- Carrots (1 cup, sliced)
- Coconut Aminos (2 tbsp)
- Fresh Basil (1 tbsp, chopped)
- Fresh Thyme (1 tbsp, chopped)
- Coconut Oil (2 tbsp)

DIRECTION

01   Preheat oven to 375°F (190°C).

02   Place salmon fillets on a baking sheet and bake for 15 minutes until cooked through.

03   In a skillet, heat coconut oil over medium heat.

04   Add cauliflower rice, broccoli, and carrots.

05   Sauté until tender, about 10 minutes.

06   Drizzle with coconut aminos and serve with salmon.

NUTRITIONAL INFO PER SERVING

- Calories 450
- Protein   30g
- Carbs   20g
- Fat   25g
- Fiber   10g
- Sugar   5g

NOTES:

Store leftover rice and salmon separately in the fridge for up to 2 days. Reheat in a skillet or microwave before serving.

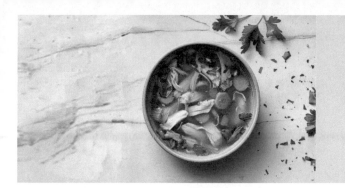

AIP CHICKEN AND VEGETABLE SOUP

INGREDIENTS

COOK TIME: 20
PREP TIME: 10
TOTAL TIME: 30
SERVINGS: 2

- Chicken Breast (2, diced)
- Carrots (1 cup, sliced)
- Celery (1 cup, sliced)
- Leeks (1 cup, sliced)
- Garlic (2 cloves, minced)
- Bone Broth (4 cups)
- Fresh Thyme (1 tsp)
- Fresh Rosemary (1 tsp)

DIRECTION

01 In a large pot, heat bone broth over medium heat.

02 Add diced chicken, carrots, celery, leeks, and garlic.

03 Stir in fresh thyme and rosemary.

04 Bring to a boil, then reduce heat and simmer for 20 minutes.

05 Season with salt and pepper to taste if desired.

06 Serve hot.

NUTRITIONAL INFO PER SERVING

- Calories 300
- Protein 25g
- Carbs 15g
- Fat 10g
- Fiber 5g
- Sugar 5g

NOTES:
Store leftovers in an airtight container in the fridge for up to 3 days. Reheat on the stove before serving.

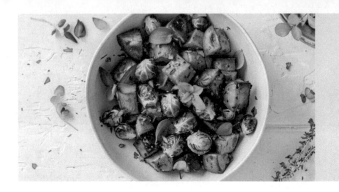

SWEET POTATO AND BRUSSELS SPROUT SALAD

INGREDIENTS

COOK TIME: 20
PREP TIME: 10
TOTAL TIME: 30
SERVINGS: 2

- Sweet Potato (2 cups, diced)
- Brussels Sprouts (2 cups, halved)
- Coconut Oil (2 tbsp)
- Fresh Rosemary (1 tsp)
- Fresh Thyme (1 tsp)
- Lemon Juice (2 tbsp)
- Salt (to taste)
- Pepper (to taste, optional)

DIRECTION

01 Preheat oven to 400°F (200°C).

02 Toss sweet potatoes and Brussels sprouts with coconut oil, rosemary, and thyme.

03 Spread on a baking sheet and roast for 20 minutes until tender.

04 Drizzle with lemon juice.

05 Season with salt and pepper to taste.

06 Serve warm or at room temperature.

NUTRITIONAL INFO PER SERVING

- Calories 350
- Protein 6g
- Carbs 45g
- Fat 20g
- Fiber 10g
- Sugar 10g

NOTES:
Store leftovers in an airtight container in the fridge for up to 2 days. Reheat in the oven or enjoy cold.

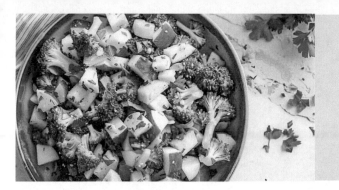

BROCCOLI AND APPLE SALAD WITH COCONUT AMINOS DRESSING

INGREDIENTS

COOK TIME: 0
PREP TIME: 10
TOTAL TIME: 10
SERVINGS: 2

- Broccoli (2 cups, florets)
- Apple (1, diced)
- Coconut Aminos (2 tbsp)
- Lemon Juice (2 tbsp)
- Fresh Parsley (2 tbsp, chopped)
- Salt (to taste)
- Pepper (to taste, optional)

DIRECTION

01 In a large bowl, combine broccoli florets and diced apple.

02 In a small bowl, mix coconut aminos, lemon juice, and fresh parsley.

03 Pour dressing over salad and toss to combine.

04 Season with salt and pepper to taste.

05 Serve immediately.

NUTRITIONAL INFO PER SERVING

- Calories 200
- Protein 4g
- Carbs 25g
- Fat 10g
- Fiber 7g
- Sugar 10g

NOTES:

Best served fresh. Store leftovers in an airtight container in the fridge for up to 2 days.

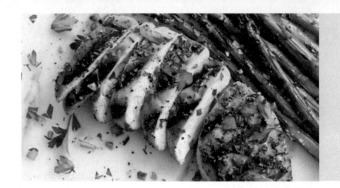

GRILLED CHICKEN AND ASPARAGUS SALAD

INGREDIENTS

COOK TIME: 15   TOTAL TIME: 25
PREP TIME: 10   SERVINGS: 2

- Chicken Breast (2)
- Asparagus (1 bunch, trimmed)
- Coconut Oil (2 tbsp)
- Lemon Juice (2 tbsp)
- Fresh Thyme (1 tsp)
- Fresh Rosemary (1 tsp)
- Salt (to taste)
- Pepper (to taste, optional)

DIRECTION

01   Preheat grill to medium-high heat.

02   Brush chicken and asparagus with coconut oil.

03   Grill chicken for 6-7 minutes per side until cooked through.

04   Grill asparagus for 3-4 minutes until tender.

05   Slice chicken and serve with grilled asparagus.

06   Drizzle with lemon juice, thyme, and rosemary.

NUTRITIONAL INFO PER SERVING

- Calories   350
- Protein   30g
- Carbs   10g
- Fat   20g
- Fiber   6g
- Sugar   2g

NOTES:

Best served fresh. Store leftovers in an airtight container in the fridge for up to 2 days. Reheat in a skillet before serving.

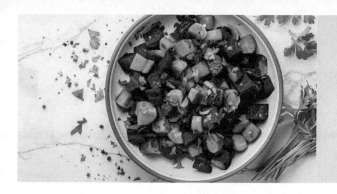

ROASTED BEET AND CARROT SALAD WITH FRESH PARSLEY

INGREDIENTS

COOK TIME: 20
PREP TIME: 10
TOTAL TIME: 30
SERVINGS: 2

- Beets (2 cups, diced)
- Carrots (1 cup, sliced)
- Coconut Oil (2 tbsp)
- Fresh Parsley (2 tbsp, chopped)
- Lemon Juice (2 tbsp)
- Salt (to taste)
- Pepper (to taste, optional)

DIRECTION

01 Preheat oven to 400°F (200°C).

02 Toss diced beets and sliced carrots with coconut oil.

03 Spread on a baking sheet and roast for 20 minutes until tender.

04 Transfer to a bowl and let cool slightly.

05 Add fresh parsley and lemon juice.

06 Season with salt and pepper to taste.

NUTRITIONAL INFO PER SERVING

- Calories   300
- Protein   5g
- Carbs   30g
- Fat   15g
- Fiber   10g
- Sugar   15g

NOTES:

Store leftovers in an airtight container in the fridge for up to 2 days. Enjoy cold or at room temperature.

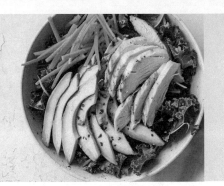

TURKEY AND KALE SALAD WITH FRESH LEMON DRESSING

INGREDIENTS

COOK TIME: 0   TOTAL TIME: 10
PREP TIME: 10   SERVINGS: 2

- 4 oz Turkey (cooked, sliced)
- 4 cups Kale (chopped)
- 1 Avocado (sliced)
- 1/2 cup Carrots (shredded)
- 1 Lemon (juiced)
- 2 tbsp Olive oil
- 1/2 tsp Sea salt
- 1/4 tsp Black pepper (optional)

DIRECTION

01 Combine kale, avocado, and shredded carrots in a bowl.

02 Whisk together lemon juice, olive oil, salt, and black pepper (optional) for dressing.

03 Toss salad with dressing.

04 Top with sliced turkey.

05 Serve immediately.

NUTRITIONAL INFO PER SERVING

- Calories   450
- Protein   22g
- Carbs   25g
- Fat   28g
- Fiber   8g
- Sugar   4g

NOTES:
Store salad and dressing separately in the fridge for up to 2 days. Add dressing just before serving.

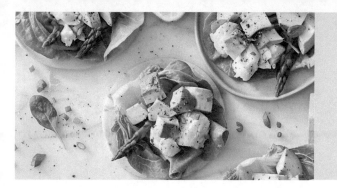

COD AND ASPARAGUS GRAIN-FREE TACOS

INGREDIENTS

COOK TIME: 10   TOTAL TIME: 20
PREP TIME: 10   SERVINGS: 2

- 4 oz Cod (cooked, flaked)
- 1/4 cup Fresh cilantro (chopped)
- 1/2 Avocado (sliced)
- 4 Lettuce leaves
- 1 Lime (quartered)
- 8 Asparagus spears (grilled, chopped)

- 1/4 tsp Sea salt
- 1/4 tsp Black pepper (optional)

DIRECTION

01 Grill asparagus until tender, then chop.

02 Flake the cooked cod.

03 Assemble tacos using lettuce leaves as shells.

04 Fill with cod, asparagus, and avocado slices.

05 Sprinkle with cilantro, salt, and pepper (optional).

06 Serve with lime wedges.

NUTRITIONAL INFO PER SERVING

- Calories   200
- Protein   20g
- Carbs   14g
- Fat   8g
- Fiber   6g
- Sugar   2g

NOTES:

Store components separately in the fridge for up to 2 days. Assemble tacos just before serving.

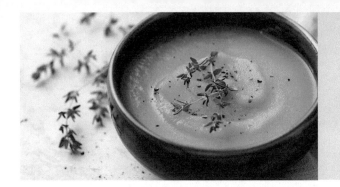

BUTTERNUT SQUASH SOUP
(FOR REINTRODUCTION)

INGREDIENTS

COOK TIME: 30   TOTAL TIME: 40
PREP TIME: 10   SERVINGS: 2

- 2 cups Butternut squash (diced)
- 1/2 Onion (diced)
- 2 cups Bone broth
- 1 cup Coconut milk
- 1 tbsp Olive oil
- 1/2 tsp Sea salt
- 1/4 tsp Black pepper (optional)
- 1/4 tsp Fresh thyme

DIRECTION

01   Heat olive oil in a pot over medium heat.

02   Add onion and sauté until translucent.

03   Add butternut squash, bone broth, salt, pepper (optional), and thyme.

04   Bring to a boil, then simmer until squash is tender.

05   Blend until smooth.

06   Stir in coconut milk and heat through.

NUTRITIONAL INFO PER SERVING

- Calories   300
- Protein   4g
- Carbs   28g
- Fat   20g
- Fiber   5g
- Sugar   6g

NOTES:
Store in an airtight container in the fridge for up to 3 days. Reheat before serving.

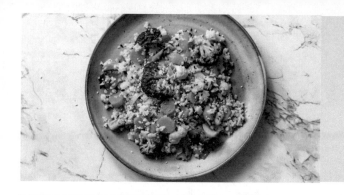

CAULIFLOWER RICE AND VEGGIE STIR-FRY WITH FRESH BASIL

INGREDIENTS

COOK TIME: 10   TOTAL TIME: 20
PREP TIME: 10   SERVINGS: 2

- 2 cups Cauliflower rice
- 1 cup Broccoli (chopped)
- 1 cup Carrots (sliced)
- 1 Zucchini (sliced)
- 1/2 Onion (sliced)
- 2 tbsp Olive oil
- 1/2 cup Fresh basil (chopped)
- 1/2 tsp Sea salt
- 1/4 tsp Black pepper (optional)

DIRECTION

01   Heat olive oil in a skillet over medium heat.

02   Add onion and cook until translucent.

03   Add broccoli, carrots, and zucchini; cook until tender.

04   Add cauliflower rice and cook for 5 minutes.

05   Stir in fresh basil, salt, and pepper (optional).

06   Serve hot.

NUTRITIONAL INFO PER SERVING

- Calories   180
- Protein   4g
- Carbs   22g
- Fat   10g
- Fiber   7g
- Sugar   6g

NOTES:

Store in an airtight container in the fridge for up to 2 days. Reheat in a skillet before serving.

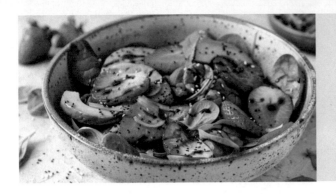

SPINACH AND STRAWBERRY SALAD WITH AVOCADO

INGREDIENTS

COOK TIME: 0
PREP TIME: 10

TOTAL TIME: 10
SERVINGS: 2

- 4 cups Spinach (chopped)
- 1 cup Strawberries (sliced)
- 1 Avocado (sliced)
- 1/4 cup Red onion (sliced)
- 2 tbsp Olive oil
- 1 tbsp Balsamic vinegar (AIP compliant)
- 1/2 tsp Sea salt
- 1/4 tsp Black pepper (optional)

DIRECTION

01 Combine spinach, strawberries, avocado, and red onion in a bowl.

02 Whisk together olive oil, balsamic vinegar, salt, and black pepper (optional).

03 Toss salad with dressing.

04 Serve immediately.

NUTRITIONAL INFO PER SERVING

- Calories 300
- Protein 4g
- Carbs 26g
- Fat 22g
- Fiber 8g
- Sugar 10g

NOTES:
Store salad and dressing separately in the fridge for up to 2 days. Add dressing just before serving.

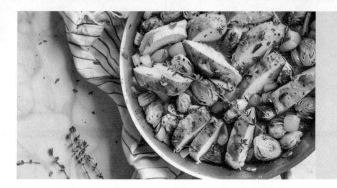

BRUSSELS SPROUTS AND TURKEY SKILLET

INGREDIENTS

COOK TIME: 15
PREP TIME: 10
TOTAL TIME: 25
SERVINGS: 2

- 6 oz Turkey (cooked, sliced)
- 2 cups Brussels sprouts (halved)
- 1/2 Onion (sliced)
- 1 tbsp Olive oil
- 1/2 tsp Sea salt
- 1/4 tsp Black pepper (optional)
- 1/4 tsp Fresh thyme

DIRECTION

01 Heat olive oil in a skillet over medium heat.

02 Add onion and cook until translucent.

03 Add Brussels sprouts and cook until tender.

04 Add cooked turkey, salt, pepper (optional), and thyme.

05 Cook until heated through.

06 Serve hot.

NUTRITIONAL INFO PER SERVING

- Calories   280
- Protein   22g
- Carbs   18g
- Fat   12g
- Fiber   6g
- Sugar   4g

NOTES:

Store in an airtight container in the fridge for up to 2 days. Reheat in a skillet before serving.

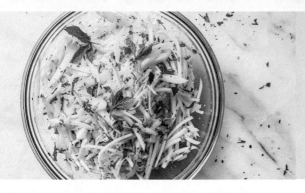

GREEN CABBAGE AND APPLE SLAW WITH FRESH MINT

INGREDIENTS

COOK TIME: 0
PREP TIME: 10
TOTAL TIME: 10
SERVINGS: 2

- 2 cups Green cabbage (shredded)
- 1 Apple (julienned)
- 1/4 cup Fresh mint (chopped)
- 1 Lemon (juiced)
- 2 tbsp Olive oil
- 1/2 tsp Sea salt
- 1/4 tsp Black pepper (optional)

DIRECTION

01 Combine cabbage, apple, and mint in a bowl.

02 Whisk together lemon juice, olive oil, salt, and black pepper (optional).

03 Toss slaw with dressing.

04 Serve immediately.

NUTRITIONAL INFO PER SERVING

- Calories   150
- Protein   1g
- Carbs   20g
- Fat   8g
- Fiber   6g
- Sugar   12g

NOTES:
Store slaw and dressing separately in the fridge for up to 1 day. Add dressing just before serving.

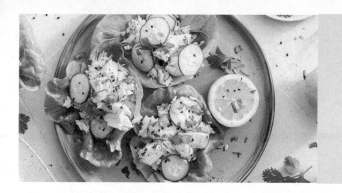

TILAPIA AND CUCUMBER WRAPS

(REINTRODUCTION: WHITE RICE)

INGREDIENTS

COOK TIME: 10
PREP TIME: 10
TOTAL TIME: 20
SERVINGS: 2

- 2 Tilapia fillets
- 1 Cucumber (sliced)
- 1 cup White rice (cooked)
- 2 Lettuce leaves
- 1 Lemon (juiced)
- 2 tbsp Fresh cilantro (chopped)
- 1 tbsp Olive oil
- 1/2 tsp Sea salt
- 1/4 tsp Black pepper (optional)

DIRECTION

01 Cook tilapia in olive oil until opaque and flaky.

02 Slice cucumber.

03 Warm white rice.

04 Layer tilapia, rice, and cucumber slices in lettuce leaves.

05 Drizzle with lemon juice, sprinkle with cilantro, salt, and pepper (optional).

06 Serve immediately.

NUTRITIONAL INFO PER SERVING

- Calories 350
- Protein 24g
- Carbs 38g
- Fat 12g
- Fiber 2g
- Sugar 3g

NOTES:
Store components separately in the fridge for up to 2 days. Assemble just before serving.

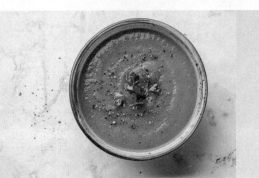

SWEET POTATO AND CARROT SOUP

INGREDIENTS

COOK TIME: 25
PREP TIME: 10

TOTAL TIME: 35
SERVINGS: 2

- 2 Sweet potatoes (diced)
- 2 Carrots (sliced)
- 1 Onion (diced)
- 2 cups Bone broth
- 1 tbsp Olive oil
- 1/2 tsp Sea salt
- 1/4 tsp Turmeric
- 1/4 tsp Ginger

DIRECTION

01 Heat olive oil in a pot over medium heat.

02 Add onion and cook until translucent.

03 Add sweet potatoes, carrots, bone broth, salt, turmeric, and ginger.

04 Bring to a boil, then simmer until vegetables are tender.

05 Blend until smooth.

06 Serve hot.

NUTRITIONAL INFO PER SERVING

- Calories 200
- Protein 4g
- Carbs 35g
- Fat 5g
- Fiber 6g
- Sugar 10g

NOTES:
Store in an airtight container in the fridge for up to 3 days. Reheat on the stovetop before serving.

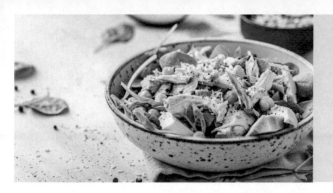

AVOCADO AND CHICKEN SALAD

(REINTRODUCTION: CHICKPEAS)

COOK TIME: 0	TOTAL TIME: 10
PREP TIME: 10	SERVINGS: 2

INGREDIENTS

- 1 Avocado (diced)
- 1 cup Chicken (cooked, shredded)
- 1/2 cup Chickpeas (rinsed)
- 2 cups Spinach (chopped)
- 1 Lemon (juiced)
- 2 tbsp Olive oil
- 1/2 tsp Sea salt
- 1/4 tsp Black pepper (optional)

DIRECTION

01 In a bowl, combine avocado, chicken, chickpeas, and spinach.

02 Whisk together lemon juice, olive oil, salt, and pepper (optional).

03 Toss salad with dressing.

04 Serve immediately.

NUTRITIONAL INFO PER SERVING

- Calories   400
- Protein   24g
- Carbs   26g
- Fat   24g
- Fiber   8g
- Sugar   2g

NOTES:

Best served immediately. Store leftovers in an airtight container in the fridge for up to 2 days.

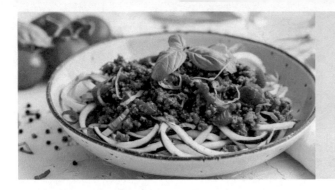

ZUCCHINI NOODLES WITH FRESH BASIL AND BEEF

(REINTRODUCTION: TOMATOES)

INGREDIENTS

COOK TIME: 15
PREP TIME: 10

TOTAL TIME: 25
SERVINGS: 2

- 1 Zucchini (spiralized)
- 8 oz Ground beef
- 1 Onion (diced)
- 2 Garlic cloves (minced)
- 2 tbsp Fresh basil (chopped)
- 1 cup Cherry tomatoes (halved, for reintroduction)
- 1 tbsp Olive oil
- 1/2 tsp Sea salt
- 1/4 tsp Black pepper (optional)

DIRECTION

01 Heat olive oil in a skillet over medium heat.

02 Add onion and garlic; cook until fragrant.

03 Add ground beef; cook until browned.

04 Add cherry tomatoes; cook until tender.

05 Stir in zucchini noodles, basil, salt, and pepper (optional).

06 Cook for 2-3 minutes and serve hot.

NUTRITIONAL INFO PER SERVING

- Calories 300
- Protein 26g
- Carbs 14g
- Fat 18g
- Fiber 4g
- Sugar 6g

NOTES:

Store in an airtight container in the fridge for up to 2 days. Reheat in a skillet before serving.

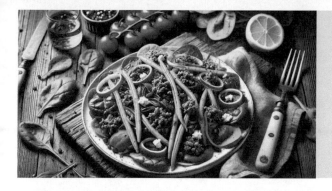

GREEN BEAN AND BEEF SALAD

(REINTRODUCTION: GREEN BEANS)

INGREDIENTS

COOK TIME: 10
PREP TIME: 10
TOTAL TIME: 20
SERVINGS: 2

- 2 cups Green beans (trimmed)
- 8 oz Beef (cooked, sliced)
- 2 cups Spinach (chopped)
- 1/2 Onion (sliced)
- 1 Lemon (juiced)
- 2 tbsp Olive oil
- 1/2 tsp Sea salt
- 1/4 tsp Black pepper (optional)
- 1 tbsp Fresh parsley (chopped)

DIRECTION

01 Steam green beans until tender.

02 In a bowl, combine green beans, beef, spinach, and onion.

03 Whisk together lemon juice, olive oil, salt, and pepper (optional).

04 Toss salad with dressing.

05 Sprinkle with parsley and serve.

NUTRITIONAL INFO PER SERVING

- Calories   350
- Protein   28g
- Carbs   14g
- Fat   22g
- Fiber   4g
- Sugar   4g

NOTES:

Best served immediately. Store leftovers in an airtight container in the fridge for up to 2 days.

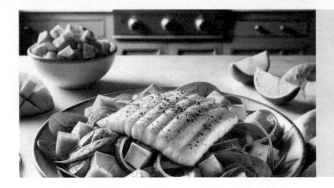

TILAPIA AND MANGO SALAD

INGREDIENTS

COOK TIME: 10   TOTAL TIME: 20
PREP TIME: 10   SERVINGS: 2

- 2 Tilapia fillets
- 1 Mango (diced)
- 1 Avocado (diced)
- 1/2 Red onion (diced)
- 2 cups Spinach (chopped)
- 1 Lime (juiced)
- 2 tbsp Olive oil
- 1/2 tsp Sea salt
- 1/4 tsp Black pepper (optional)

DIRECTION

01 Cook tilapia in olive oil until opaque and flaky.

02 In a bowl, combine mango, avocado, red onion, and spinach.

03 Whisk together lime juice, olive oil, salt, and pepper (optional).

04 Toss salad with dressing.

05 Top with cooked tilapia and serve.

NUTRITIONAL INFO PER SERVING

- Calories   350
- Protein   28g
- Carbs   22g
- Fat   18g
- Fiber   6g
- Sugar   8g

NOTES:

Best served immediately. Store leftovers in an airtight container in the fridge for up to 2 days.

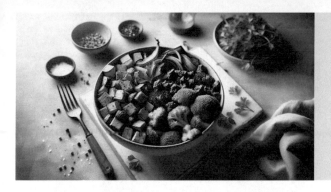

BROCCOLI AND BEEF POWER BOWL

INGREDIENTS

COOK TIME: 20
PREP TIME: 10
TOTAL TIME: 30
SERVINGS: 2

- 2 cups Broccoli (chopped)
- 8 oz Ground beef
- 1 Sweet potato (diced)
- 1 Onion (diced)
- 1 tbsp Olive oil
- 1/2 tsp Sea salt
- 1/4 tsp Black pepper (optional)
- 1 tbsp Fresh parsley (chopped)

DIRECTION

01 Preheat oven to 375°F (190°C).

02 Toss sweet potato with olive oil, salt, and pepper (optional).

03 Spread on a baking sheet and roast for 20 minutes.

04 Cook ground beef and onion in a skillet until browned.

05 Steam broccoli until tender.

06 Combine sweet potato, beef, and broccoli in bowls. Top with parsley.

NUTRITIONAL INFO PER SERVING

- Calories 400
- Protein 30g
- Carbs 30g
- Fat 18g
- Fiber 8g
- Sugar 6g

NOTES:
Store components separately in the fridge for up to 2 days. Reheat before serving.

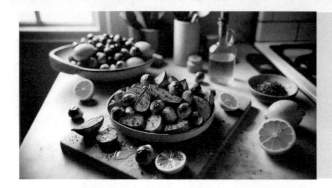

SWEET POTATO AND BRUSSELS SPROUTS SALAD WITH LEMON DRESSING

INGREDIENTS

COOK TIME: 30
PREP TIME: 10
TOTAL TIME: 40
SERVINGS: 2

- 2 Sweet potatoes (diced)
- 2 cups Brussels sprouts (halved)
- 1 Lemon (juiced)
- 2 tbsp Olive oil
- 1 tbsp Honey
- 1/2 tsp Sea salt
- 1/4 tsp Black pepper (optional)
- 1 tbsp Fresh parsley (chopped)

DIRECTION

01   Preheat oven to 400°F (200°C).

02   Toss sweet potatoes and Brussels sprouts with 1 tbsp olive oil, salt, and pepper (optional).

03   Roast for 30 minutes, until tender.

04   In a bowl, whisk lemon juice, remaining olive oil, honey, and parsley.

05   Toss roasted vegetables with dressing.

06   Serve warm or at room temperature.

NUTRITIONAL INFO PER SERVING

- Calories   250
- Protein   4g
- Carbs   45g
- Fat   8g
- Fiber   8g
- Sugar   14g

NOTES:

Store in an airtight container in the fridge for up to 2 days. Reheat before serving.

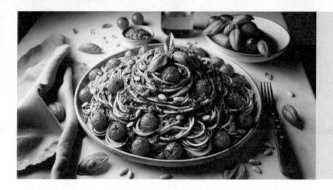

ZUCCHINI NOODLES WITH PESTO AND CHERRY TOMATOES
(FOR REINTRODUCTION)

INGREDIENTS

COOK TIME: 0
PREP TIME: 15
TOTAL TIME: 15
SERVINGS: 2

- 2 Zucchini (spiralized)
- 1 cup Cherry tomatoes (halved)
- 1 cup Fresh basil
- 1/4 cup Olive oil
- 2 tbsp Pine nuts (optional)
- 2 Garlic cloves
- 1/4 tsp Sea salt
- 1/4 tsp Black pepper (optional)
- 1 tbsp Lemon juice
- 1/4 cup Nutritional yeast

DIRECTION

01   Spiralize zucchini.

02   In a blender, combine basil, olive oil, pine nuts (optional), garlic, sea salt, pepper (optional), lemon juice, and nutritional yeast to make pesto.

03   Toss zucchini noodles with pesto.

04   Add cherry tomatoes.

05   Serve immediately.

NUTRITIONAL INFO PER SERVING

- Calories   300
- Protein   8g
- Carbs   20g
- Fat   22g
- Fiber   4g
- Sugar   10g

NOTES:

Best served immediately. Store pesto in an airtight container in the fridge for up to 3 days.

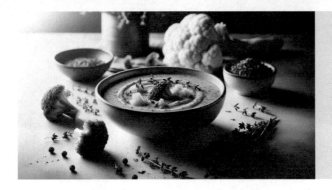

BROCCOLI AND CAULIFLOWER SOUP WITH FRESH THYME

INGREDIENTS

COOK TIME: 20
PREP TIME: 10
TOTAL TIME: 30
SERVINGS: 2

- 2 cups Broccoli (chopped)
- 2 cups Cauliflower (chopped)
- 1 Onion (diced)
- 2 Garlic cloves (minced)
- 2 cups Bone broth
- 1 tbsp Olive oil
- 1/2 tsp Sea salt
- 1/4 tsp Black pepper (optional)
- 1 tbsp Fresh thyme (chopped)

DIRECTION

01   Heat olive oil in a pot over medium heat.

02   Add onion and garlic; cook until translucent.

03   Add broccoli, cauliflower, bone broth, salt, and pepper (optional).

04   Bring to a boil, then simmer until vegetables are tender.

05   Blend until smooth.

06   Stir in fresh thyme and serve hot.

NUTRITIONAL INFO PER SERVING

- Calories   200
- Protein   4g
- Carbs   20g
- Fat   12g
- Fiber   6g
- Sugar   6g

NOTES:
Store in an airtight container in the fridge for up to 3 days. Reheat before serving.

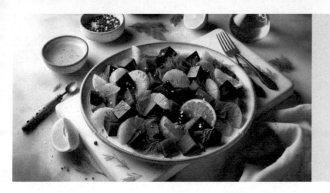

BEET AND ORANGE SALAD WITH FRESH DILL

INGREDIENTS

COOK TIME: 0
PREP TIME: 10
TOTAL TIME: 10
SERVINGS: 2

- 2 Beets (cooked, diced)
- 2 Oranges (segmented)
- 1 tbsp Fresh dill (chopped)
- 2 tbsp Olive oil
- 1 tbsp Lemon juice
- 1/2 tsp Sea salt
- 1/4 tsp Black pepper (optional)

DIRECTION

01 Cook and dice beets.

02 Segment oranges.

03 In a bowl, whisk olive oil, lemon juice, sea salt, and pepper (optional).

04 Toss beets and oranges with dressing.

05 Sprinkle with fresh dill.

06 Serve immediately.

NUTRITIONAL INFO PER SERVING

- Calories   180
- Protein   2g
- Carbs   30g
- Fat   8g
- Fiber   8g
- Sugar   20g

NOTES:
Best served immediately. Store in an airtight container in the fridge for up to 1 day.

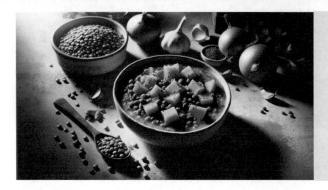

BUTTERNUT SQUASH AND LENTIL STEW

(FOR REINTRODUCTION)

INGREDIENTS

COOK TIME: 30
PREP TIME: 10

TOTAL TIME: 40
SERVINGS: 2

- 2 cups Butternut squash (diced)
- 1 cup Lentils (cooked)
- 1 Onion (diced)
- 2 Garlic cloves (minced)
- 2 cups Bone broth
- 1 tbsp Olive oil
- 1/2 tsp Sea salt
- 1/4 tsp Black pepper (optional)
- 1 tbsp Fresh parsley (chopped)

DIRECTION

01   Heat olive oil in a pot over medium heat.

02   Add onion and garlic; cook until translucent.

03   Add butternut squash, lentils, bone broth, salt, and pepper (optional).

04   Bring to a boil, then simmer until squash is tender.

05   Stir in fresh parsley and serve hot.

NUTRITIONAL INFO PER SERVING

- Calories   300
- Protein   10g
- Carbs   45g
- Fat   10g
- Fiber   12g
- Sugar   10g

NOTES:

Store in an airtight container in the fridge for up to 3 days. Reheat before serving.

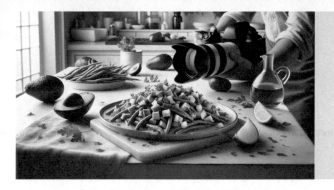

AVOCADO AND GREEN BEAN SALAD WITH FRESH PARSLEY
(FOR REINTRODUCTION)

INGREDIENTS

COOK TIME: 5
PREP TIME: 10
TOTAL TIME: 15
SERVINGS: 2

- 1 Avocado (diced)
- 1 cup Green beans (blanched)
- 1/2 Onion (diced)
- 1 Lemon (juiced)
- 2 tbsp Olive oil
- 1/4 tsp Sea salt
- 1/4 tsp Black pepper (optional)
- 1 tbsp Fresh parsley (chopped)

DIRECTION

01 Blanch green beans.

02 In a bowl, combine diced avocado, blanched green beans, and diced onion.

03 Whisk together lemon juice, olive oil, salt, and pepper (optional).

04 Toss salad with dressing.

05 Sprinkle with fresh parsley and serve.

NUTRITIONAL INFO PER SERVING

- Calories   250
- Protein   4g
- Carbs   18g
- Fat   20g
- Fiber   10g
- Sugar   4g

NOTES:

Best served immediately. Store leftovers in an airtight container in the fridge for up to 1 day.

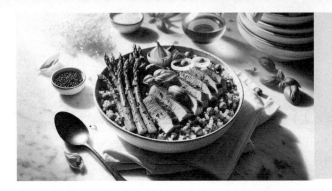

PORK AND ASPARAGUS QUINOA BOWL

(FOR REINTRODUCTION)

INGREDIENTS

COOK TIME: 10
PREP TIME: 10
TOTAL TIME: 20
SERVINGS: 2

- 8 oz Pork (cooked, sliced)
- 1 cup Quinoa (cooked)
- 1 bunch Asparagus (trimmed, cooked)
- 1/2 Onion (sliced)
- 1 tbsp Olive oil
- 1 Lemon (juiced)
- 1/4 tsp Sea salt
- 1/4 tsp Black pepper (optional)
- 1 tbsp Fresh basil (chopped)

DIRECTION

01 Cook quinoa according to package instructions.

02 Cook and slice pork.

03 Trim and cook asparagus.

04 In a bowl, combine quinoa, pork, asparagus, and sliced onion.

05 Whisk together olive oil, lemon juice, salt, and pepper (optional).

06 Toss bowl ingredients with dressing, sprinkle with fresh basil, and serve.

NUTRITIONAL INFO PER SERVING

- Calories 450
- Protein 35g
- Carbs 35g
- Fat 18g
- Fiber 8g
- Sugar 6g

NOTES:

Store components separately in the fridge for up to 2 days. Reheat before serving.

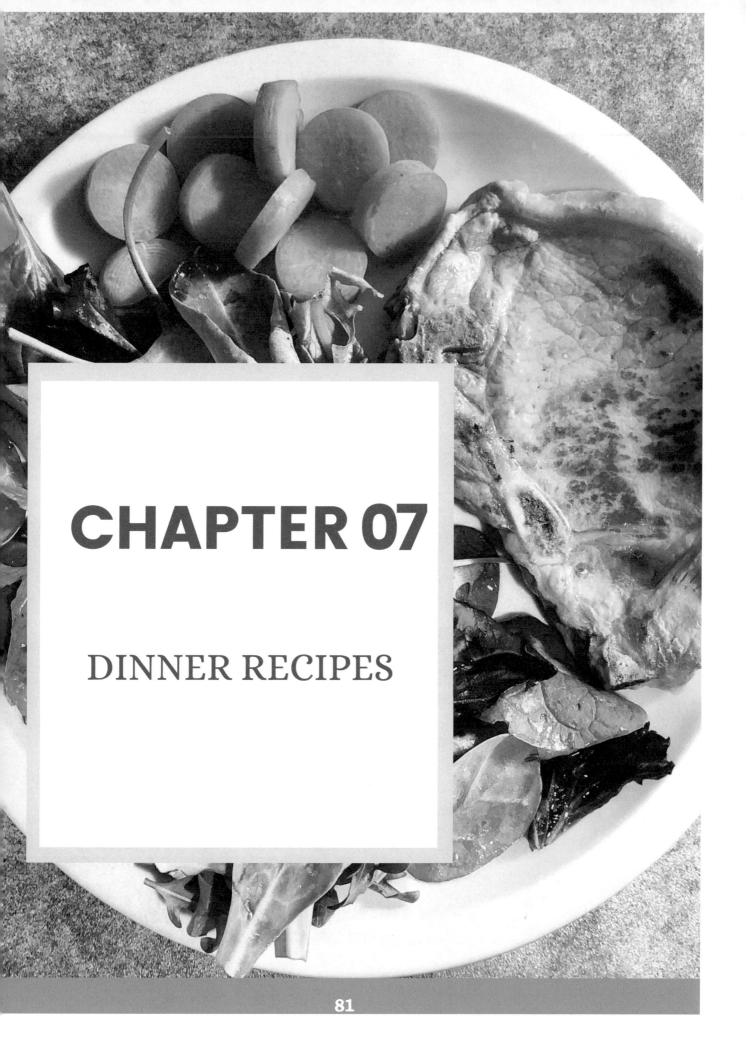

CHAPTER 07

DINNER RECIPES

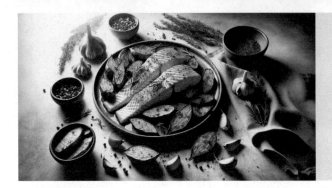

BAKED SALMON WITH GARLIC AND HERB SWEET POTATOES

INGREDIENTS

COOK TIME: 20
PREP TIME: 10

TOTAL TIME: 30
SERVINGS: 2

- Salmon (2 fillets)
- Sweet Potatoes (2 cups, diced)
- Garlic (2 cloves, minced)
- Fresh Rosemary (1 tsp)
- Fresh Thyme (1 tsp)
- Coconut Oil (2 tbsp)
- Salt (to taste)
- Pepper (to taste, optional)

DIRECTION

01 Preheat oven to 375°F (190°C).

02 Toss sweet potatoes with coconut oil, garlic, rosemary, and thyme.

03 Spread sweet potatoes on a baking sheet and bake for 20 minutes.

04 Place salmon fillets on another baking sheet.

05 Bake salmon for 15 minutes until cooked through.

06 Serve salmon with roasted sweet potatoes.

NUTRITIONAL INFO PER SERVING

- Calories   400
- Protein   30g
- Carbs   30g
- Fat   20g
- Fiber   6g
- Sugar   5g

NOTES:
Store leftovers in an airtight container in the fridge for up to 2 days. Reheat in oven or skillet before serving.

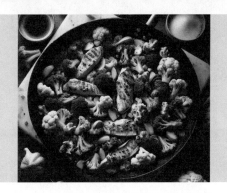

CHICKEN STIR-FRY WITH BROCCOLI AND CAULIFLOWER

INGREDIENTS

COOK TIME: 15 TOTAL TIME: 25
PREP TIME: 10 SERVINGS: 2

- Chicken Breast (2, sliced)
- Broccoli (2 cups, florets)
- Cauliflower (2 cups, florets)
- Garlic (2 cloves, minced)
- Coconut Aminos (2 tbsp)
- Coconut Oil (2 tbsp)
- Fresh Ginger (1 tsp, grated)
- Salt (to taste)
- Pepper (to taste, optional)

DIRECTION

01 Heat coconut oil in a large skillet over medium heat.

02 Add sliced chicken and cook until browned, about 5 minutes.

03 Add broccoli, cauliflower, garlic, and ginger.

04 Sauté until vegetables are tender, about 10 minutes.

05 Stir in coconut aminos and cook for another 2 minutes.

06 Serve hot.

NUTRITIONAL INFO PER SERVING

- Calories   350
- Protein   30g
- Carbs   15g
- Fat   20g
- Fiber   6g
- Sugar   5g

NOTES:

Store leftovers in an airtight container in the fridge for up to 2 days. Reheat in a skillet or microwave before serving.

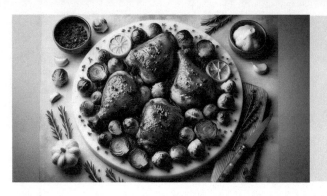

GARLIC AND HERB ROASTED CHICKEN WITH BRUSSELS SPROUTS

INGREDIENTS

COOK TIME: 25
PREP TIME: 10

TOTAL TIME: 35
SERVINGS: 2

- Chicken Thighs (4)
- Brussels Sprouts (2 cups, halved)
- Garlic (4 cloves, minced)
- Fresh Rosemary (1 tsp)
- Fresh Thyme (1 tsp)
- Coconut Oil (2 tbsp)
- Lemon Juice (2 tbsp)
- Salt (to taste)
- Pepper (to taste, optional)

DIRECTION

01 Preheat oven to 400°F (200°C).

02 Toss Brussels sprouts with coconut oil, garlic, rosemary, and thyme.

03 Spread Brussels sprouts on a baking sheet and roast for 15 minutes.

04 Place chicken thighs on another baking sheet.

05 Roast chicken for 25 minutes until cooked through.

06 Drizzle chicken and Brussels sprouts with lemon juice.

NUTRITIONAL INFO PER SERVING

- Calories   450
- Protein   35g
- Carbs   20g
- Fat   25g
- Fiber   8g
- Sugar   5g

NOTES:

Store leftovers in an airtight container in the fridge for up to 2 days. Reheat in oven or skillet before serving.

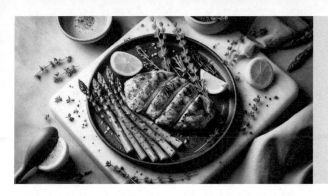

GRILLED LEMON HERB CHICKEN WITH ASPARAGUS

INGREDIENTS

COOK TIME: 15	TOTAL TIME: 25
PREP TIME: 10	SERVINGS: 2

- Chicken Breast (2)
- Asparagus (1 bunch, trimmed)
- Lemon Juice (2 tbsp)
- Fresh Rosemary (1 tsp)
- Fresh Thyme (1 tsp)
- Coconut Oil (2 tbsp)
- Salt (to taste)
- Pepper (to taste, optional)

DIRECTION

01   Preheat grill to medium-high heat.

02   Brush chicken and asparagus with coconut oil.

03   Grill chicken for 6-7 minutes per side until cooked through.

04   Grill asparagus for 3-4 minutes until tender.

05   Drizzle chicken and asparagus with lemon juice.

06   Sprinkle with rosemary and thyme before serving.

NUTRITIONAL INFO PER SERVING

- Calories   350
- Protein   30g
- Carbs   10g
- Fat   20g
- Fiber   6g
- Sugar   2g

NOTES:

Best served fresh. Store leftovers in an airtight container in the fridge for up to 2 days. Reheat in a skillet before serving.

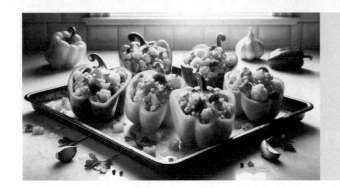

CAULIFLOWER RICE STUFFED PEPPERS

INGREDIENTS

COOK TIME: 20
PREP TIME: 15
TOTAL TIME: 35
SERVINGS: 2

- Bell Peppers (2, halved)
- Cauliflower (2 cups, riced)
- Chicken Breast (1, diced)
- Garlic (2 cloves, minced)
- Fresh Parsley (2 tbsp)
- Coconut Oil (2 tbsp)
- Coconut Aminos (2 tbsp)
- Salt (to taste)
- Pepper (to taste, optional)

DIRECTION

01   Preheat oven to 375°F (190°C).

02   Heat coconut oil in a skillet over medium heat.

03   Add diced chicken and cook until browned, about 5 minutes.

04   Add cauliflower rice, garlic, and coconut aminos.

05   Sauté until cauliflower is tender, about 10 minutes.

06   Fill bell pepper halves with the mixture.

NUTRITIONAL INFO PER SERVING

- Calories   300
- Protein   25g
- Carbs   20g
- Fat   15g
- Fiber   8g
- Sugar   5g

NOTES:

Store leftovers in an airtight container in the fridge for up to 2 days. Reheat in the oven or microwave before serving.

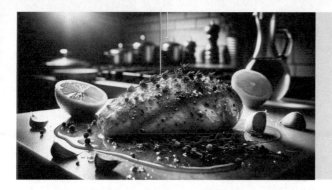

BAKED CHICKEN WITH LEMON AND FRESH THYME

INGREDIENTS

COOK TIME: 20
PREP TIME: 10
TOTAL TIME: 30
SERVINGS: 2

- Chicken Breast (2)
- Lemon Juice (2 tbsp)
- Fresh Thyme (2 tsp)
- Garlic (2 cloves, minced)
- Coconut Oil (2 tbsp)
- Salt (to taste)
- Pepper (to taste, optional)

DIRECTION

01 Preheat oven to 375°F (190°C).

02 In a small bowl, mix lemon juice, fresh thyme, and minced garlic.

03 Rub mixture over chicken breasts.

04 Place chicken in a baking dish and drizzle with coconut oil.

05 Bake for 20 minutes until cooked through.

06 Serve hot.

NUTRITIONAL INFO PER SERVING

- Calories 300
- Protein 25g
- Carbs 10g
- Fat 15g
- Fiber 2g
- Sugar 2g

NOTES:
Store leftovers in an airtight container in the fridge for up to 2 days. Reheat in the oven or microwave before serving.

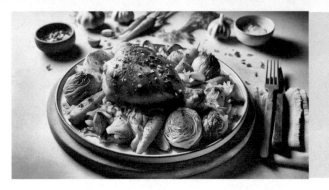

ROASTED GARLIC CHICKEN WITH CABBAGE AND CARROTS

INGREDIENTS

COOK TIME: 25
PREP TIME: 10

TOTAL TIME: 35
SERVINGS: 2

- Chicken Thighs (4)
- Cabbage (2 cups, sliced)
- Carrots (2 cups, sliced)
- Garlic (4 cloves, minced)
- Fresh Parsley (2 tbsp)
- Coconut Oil (2 tbsp)

- Salt (to taste)
- Pepper (to taste, optional)

DIRECTION

01 Preheat oven to 400°F (200°C).

02 Toss cabbage and carrots with coconut oil and garlic.

03 Spread cabbage and carrots on a baking sheet.

04 Place chicken thighs on top of vegetables.

05 Roast for 25 minutes until chicken is cooked through.

06 Sprinkle with fresh parsley before serving.

NUTRITIONAL INFO PER SERVING

- Calories   450
- Protein   35g
- Carbs   25g
- Fat   25g
- Fiber   8g
- Sugar   8g

NOTES:
Store leftovers in an airtight container in the fridge for up to 2 days. Reheat in the oven or skillet before serving.

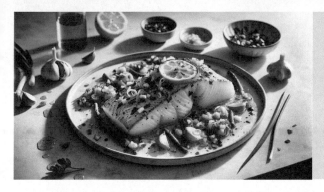

LEMON HERB COD WITH GARLIC AND GREEN ONIONS

INGREDIENTS

COOK TIME: 15
PREP TIME: 10

TOTAL TIME: 25
SERVINGS: 2

- 2 Cod fillets
- 1 Lemon (juiced, zested)
- 2 Garlic cloves (minced)
- 2 Green onions (chopped)
- 2 tbsp Olive oil
- 1/2 tsp Sea salt
- 1/4 tsp Black pepper (optional)
- 1 tbsp Fresh parsley (chopped)

DIRECTION

01 Preheat oven to 375°F (190°C).

02 Place cod fillets on a baking sheet.

03 Drizzle with olive oil, lemon juice, and zest.

04 Sprinkle with garlic, green onions, salt, pepper (optional), and parsley.

05 Bake for 15 minutes or until cooked through.

06 Serve hot.

NUTRITIONAL INFO PER SERVING

- Calories 250
- Protein 25g
- Carbs 5g
- Fat 14g
- Fiber 1g
- Sugar 1g

NOTES:

Store in an airtight container in the fridge for up to 2 days. Reheat in the oven before serving.

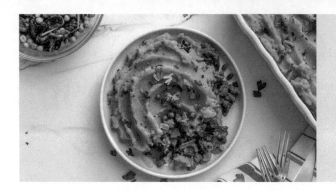

TURKEY AND SWEET POTATO SHEPHERD'S PIE

INGREDIENTS

COOK TIME: 30
PREP TIME: 15
TOTAL TIME: 45
SERVINGS: 2

- 8 oz Ground turkey
- 2 Sweet potatoes (mashed)
- 1/2 Onion (diced)
- 2 cups Spinach (chopped)
- 1/4 peas
- 2 tbsp Olive oil
- 1/2 tsp Sea salt
- 1/4 tsp Black pepper (optional)
- 1/2 cup Bone broth

DIRECTION

01 Preheat oven to 375°F (190°C).

02 Heat olive oil in a skillet over medium heat.

03 Add onion and peas, cook until tender.

04 Add ground turkey, cook until browned.

05 Stir in spinach, bone broth, salt, and pepper (optional).

06 Transfer to a baking dish, top with mashed sweet potatoes, and bake for 20 minutes.

NUTRITIONAL INFO PER SERVING

- Calories 450
- Protein 28g
- Carbs 45g
- Fat 18g
- Fiber 7g
- Sugar 7g

NOTES:

Store in an airtight container in the fridge for up to 3 days. Reheat in the oven before serving.

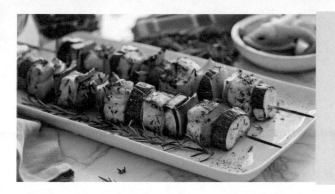

GRILLED BELL PEPPERS AND TURKEY KEBABS
(FOR REINTRODUCTION)

INGREDIENTS

COOK TIME: 10
PREP TIME: 15
TOTAL TIME: 25
SERVINGS: 2

- 6 oz Turkey (cubed)
- 2 Bell peppers (cubed)
- 1 Zucchini (sliced)
- 1 Onion (quartered)
- 1 Lemon (juiced)
- 2 tbsp Olive oil
- 1/2 tsp Sea salt
- 1/4 tsp Black pepper (optional)
- 1 tbsp Fresh rosemary (chopped)

DIRECTION

01 Preheat grill to medium-high heat.

02 In a bowl, mix lemon juice, olive oil, salt, pepper (optional), and rosemary.

03 Thread turkey, bell peppers, zucchini, and onion onto skewers.

04 Brush with marinade.

05 Grill for 10-15 minutes, turning occasionally.

06 Serve hot.

NUTRITIONAL INFO PER SERVING

- Calories   300
- Protein   25g
- Carbs   20g
- Fat   14g
- Fiber   4g
- Sugar   5g

NOTES:
Store leftovers in an airtight container in the fridge for up to 2 days. Reheat on the grill or in the oven before serving.

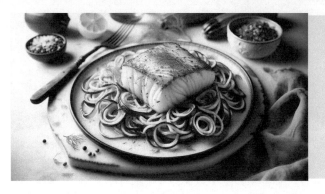

BAKED COD WITH FRESH DILL AND ZUCCHINI NOODLES

INGREDIENTS

COOK TIME: 15
PREP TIME: 10

TOTAL TIME: 25
SERVINGS: 2

- 2 Cod fillets
- 1 Zucchini (spiralized)
- 2 tbsp Fresh dill (chopped)
- 1 Lemon (juiced)
- 2 Garlic cloves (minced)
- 2 tbsp Olive oil
- 1/2 tsp Sea salt
- 1/4 tsp Black pepper (optional)

DIRECTION

01   Preheat oven to 375°F (190°C).

02   Place cod fillets on a baking sheet.

03   Drizzle with olive oil, lemon juice, garlic, salt, pepper (optional), and dill.

04   Bake for 15 minutes or until cooked through.

05   Spiralize zucchini and serve raw or lightly sautéed.

06   Serve cod over zucchini noodles.

NUTRITIONAL INFO PER SERVING

- Calories   220
- Protein   25g
- Carbs   5g
- Fat   10g
- Fiber   1g
- Sugar   2g

NOTES:

Store in an airtight container in the fridge for up to 2 days. Reheat cod in the oven before serving. Zucchini noodles can be stored raw.

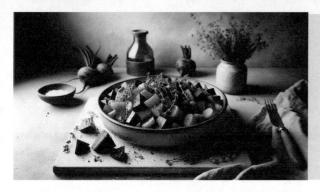

ROASTED BEETS AND CARROTS WITH FRESH THYME

INGREDIENTS

COOK TIME: 30
PREP TIME: 10

TOTAL TIME: 40
SERVINGS: 2

- 2 Beets (diced)
- 2 Carrots (diced)
- 2 tbsp Olive oil
- 1 tbsp Fresh thyme (chopped)
- 1/2 tsp Sea salt
- 1/4 tsp Black pepper (optional)

DIRECTION

01   Preheat oven to 400°F (200°C).

02   Toss beets and carrots with olive oil, thyme, salt, and pepper (optional).

03   Spread on a baking sheet.

04   Roast for 30 minutes or until tender, stirring halfway through.

05   Serve hot.

NUTRITIONAL INFO PER SERVING

- Calories   180
- Protein   2g
- Carbs   20g
- Fat   10g
- Fiber   6g
- Sugar   10g

NOTES:

Store in an airtight container in the fridge for up to 3 days. Reheat in the oven before serving.

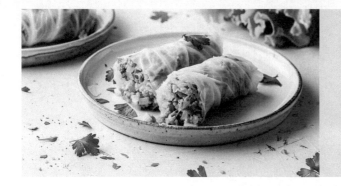

TURKEY STUFFED GREEN CABBAGE ROLLS

INGREDIENTS

COOK TIME: 30   TOTAL TIME: 45
PREP TIME: 15   SERVINGS: 2

- 8 Green cabbage leaves
- 8 oz Ground turkey
- 1/2 Onion (diced)
- 1 Carrot (diced)
- 1 cup Cauliflower rice
- 2 tbsp Olive oil
- 1/2 tsp Sea salt
- 1/4 tsp Black pepper (optional)
- 1 cup Bone broth
- 1 tbsp Fresh parsley (chopped)

DIRECTION

01   Preheat oven to 375°F (190°C).

02   Blanch cabbage leaves in boiling water for 2 minutes.

03   Heat olive oil in a skillet over medium heat.

04   Add onion and carrot, cook until tender.

05   Add ground turkey, cook until browned.

06   Mix in cauliflower rice, salt, pepper (optional), and parsley. Roll mixture into cabbage leaves and place in a baking dish. Pour bone broth over rolls and bake for 20 minutes.

NUTRITIONAL INFO PER SERVING

- Calories   350
- Protein   25g
- Carbs   20g
- Fat   16g
- Fiber   5g
- Sugar   4g

NOTES:

Store in an airtight container in the fridge for up to 2 days. Reheat in the oven before serving.

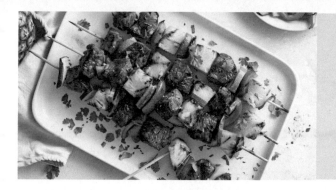

PINEAPPLE AND TURKEY STIR-FRY WITH FRESH CILANTRO

INGREDIENTS

COOK TIME: 10
PREP TIME: 10
TOTAL TIME: 20
SERVINGS: 2

- 6 oz Ground turkey
- 1 cup Pineapple (diced)
- 1 Zucchini (sliced)
- 1 Red bell pepper (sliced, for reintroduction)
- 2 Garlic cloves (minced)
- 2 tbsp Olive oil
- 1/4 cup Fresh cilantro (chopped)
- 1/2 tsp Sea salt
- 1/4 tsp Black pepper (optional)

DIRECTION

01 Heat olive oil in a skillet over medium heat.

02 Add garlic and cook until fragrant.

03 Add ground turkey and cook until browned.

04 Add pineapple, zucchini, and bell pepper; cook until tender.

05 Stir in cilantro, salt, and pepper (optional).

06 Serve hot.

NUTRITIONAL INFO PER SERVING

- Calories 320
- Protein 24g
- Carbs 25g
- Fat 14g
- Fiber 5g
- Sugar 12g

NOTES:

Store in an airtight container in the fridge for up to 2 days. Reheat in a skillet before serving.

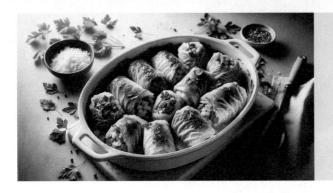

STUFFED CABBAGE ROLLS WITH BEEF

INGREDIENTS

COOK TIME: 30
PREP TIME: 15
TOTAL TIME: 45
SERVINGS: 2

- 8 Green cabbage leaves
- 8 oz Ground beef
- 1/2 Onion (diced)
- 1 Carrot (diced)
- 1 cup Cauliflower rice
- 2 tbsp Olive oil
- 1/2 tsp Sea salt
- 1/4 tsp Black pepper (optional)
- 1 cup Bone broth
- 1 tbsp Fresh parsley (chopped)

DIRECTION

01   Preheat oven to 375°F (190°C).

02   Blanch cabbage leaves in boiling water for 2 minutes.

03   Heat olive oil in a skillet over medium heat.

04   Add onion and carrot, cook until tender.

05   Add ground beef, cook until browned.

06   Mix in cauliflower rice, salt, pepper (optional), and parsley. Roll mixture into cabbage leaves and place in a baking dish. Pour bone broth over rolls and bake for 20 minutes.

NUTRITIONAL INFO PER SERVING

- Calories   350
- Protein   25g
- Carbs   20g
- Fat   16g
- Fiber   5g
- Sugar   4g

NOTES:
Store in an airtight container in the fridge for up to 2 days. Reheat in the oven before serving.

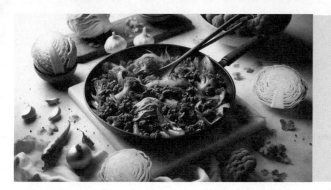

BEEF AND GREEN CABBAGE STIR-FRY

INGREDIENTS

COOK TIME: 15
PREP TIME: 10

TOTAL TIME: 25
SERVINGS: 2

- 8 oz Ground beef
- 2 cups Green cabbage (shredded)
- 1/2 Onion (sliced)
- 2 Garlic cloves (minced)
- 1 tbsp Olive oil
- 1/2 tsp Sea salt
- 1/4 tsp Black pepper (optional)
- 1 tbsp Fresh cilantro (chopped)

DIRECTION

01 Heat olive oil in a skillet over medium heat.

02 Add onion and garlic; cook until fragrant.

03 Add ground beef; cook until browned.

04 Add shredded cabbage, salt, and pepper (optional).

05 Cook until cabbage is tender.

06 Stir in fresh cilantro and serve hot.

NUTRITIONAL INFO PER SERVING

- Calories 300
- Protein 26g
- Carbs 14g
- Fat 18g
- Fiber 4g
- Sugar 3g

NOTES:

Store in an airtight container in the fridge for up to 2 days. Reheat in a skillet before serving.

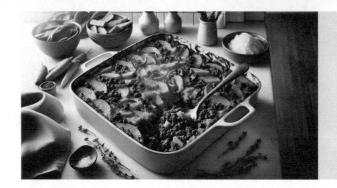

SWEET POTATO AND BEEF CASSEROLE

INGREDIENTS

COOK TIME: 30
PREP TIME: 15
TOTAL TIME: 45
SERVINGS: 2

- 2 Sweet potatoes (sliced)
- 8 oz Ground beef
- 1/2 Onion (diced)
- 1 Carrot (diced)
- 1 cup Spinach (chopped)
- 2 tbsp Olive oil
- 1/2 tsp Sea salt
- 1/4 tsp Black pepper (optional)
- 1 cup Bone broth
- 1 tbsp Fresh thyme (chopped)

DIRECTION

01 Preheat oven to 375°F (190°C).

02 Heat olive oil in a skillet over medium heat.

03 Add onion and carrot, cook until tender.

04 Add ground beef, cook until browned.

05 Layer sweet potatoes and spinach in a baking dish.

06 Pour beef mixture over, add bone broth, top with fresh thyme, and bake for 30 minutes.

NUTRITIONAL INFO PER SERVING

- Calories   450
- Protein   28g
- Carbs   45g
- Fat   18g
- Fiber   7g
- Sugar   7g

NOTES:

Store in an airtight container in the fridge for up to 3 days. Reheat in the oven before serving.

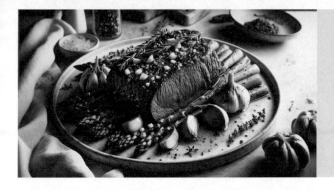

GARLIC AND HERB ROASTED BEEF WITH ASPARAGUS

INGREDIENTS

COOK TIME: 30
PREP TIME: 10
TOTAL TIME: 40
SERVINGS: 2

- 8 oz Beef (roast or steaks)
- 1 lb Asparagus (trimmed)
- 2 Garlic cloves (minced)
- 2 tbsp Olive oil
- 1 Lemon (juiced)
- 1/2 tsp Sea salt
- 1/4 tsp Black pepper (optional)
- 1 tbsp Fresh rosemary (chopped)
- 1 tbsp Fresh thyme (chopped)

DIRECTION

01 Preheat oven to 400°F (200°C).

02 Mix olive oil, garlic, lemon juice, salt, pepper (optional), rosemary, and thyme.

03 Rub mixture over beef and asparagus.

04 Place beef and asparagus on a baking sheet.

05 Roast for 30 minutes or until beef is cooked to desired doneness.

06 Serve hot.

NUTRITIONAL INFO PER SERVING

- Calories   500
- Protein   40g
- Carbs   15g
- Fat   28g
- Fiber   6g
- Sugar   4g

NOTES:
Store leftovers in an airtight container in the fridge for up to 2 days. Reheat in the oven before serving.

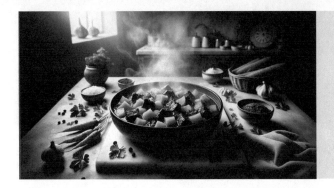

BUTTERNUT SQUASH AND BEEF STEW

(REINTRODUCTION: BUTTERNUT SQUASH)

INGREDIENTS

COOK TIME: 40
PREP TIME: 10
TOTAL TIME: 50
SERVINGS: 2

- 2 cups Butternut squash (diced)
- 8 oz Beef (cubed)
- 1 Onion (diced)
- 2 Carrots (sliced)
- 2 cups Bone broth
- 1 tbsp Olive oil
- 1/2 tsp Sea salt
- 1/4 tsp Black pepper (optional)
- 1 tbsp Fresh parsley (chopped)

DIRECTION

01 Heat olive oil in a pot over medium heat.

02 Add onion and cook until translucent.

03 Add beef and cook until browned.

04 Add butternut squash, carrots, bone broth, salt, and pepper (optional).

05 Bring to a boil, then simmer until vegetables are tender.

06 Stir in fresh parsley and serve hot.

NUTRITIONAL INFO PER SERVING

- Calories 350
- Protein 28g
- Carbs 30g
- Fat 16g
- Fiber 6g
- Sugar 6g

NOTES:
Store in an airtight container in the fridge for up to 3 days. Reheat on the stovetop before serving.

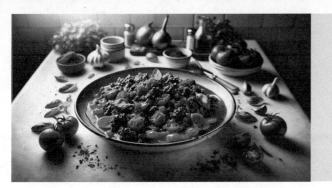

TOMATO AND BEEF RAGU

(REINTRODUCTION: TOMATOES)

INGREDIENTS

COOK TIME: 30   TOTAL TIME: 40
PREP TIME: 10   SERVINGS: 2

- 8 oz Ground beef
- 2 cups Tomatoes (diced)
- 1 Onion (diced)
- 2 Garlic cloves (minced)
- 1 Carrot (diced)
- 1 tbsp Olive oil

- 1/2 tsp Sea salt
- 1/4 tsp Black pepper (optional)
- 1 tbsp Fresh basil (chopped)
- 1 tbsp Fresh oregano (chopped)

DIRECTION

01   Heat olive oil in a skillet over medium heat.

02   Add onion, garlic, and carrot; cook until tender.

03   Add ground beef; cook until browned.

04   Add diced tomatoes, salt, and pepper (optional).

05   Simmer for 20 minutes.

06   Stir in fresh basil and oregano, and serve hot.

NUTRITIONAL INFO PER SERVING

- Calories   400
- Protein   30g
- Carbs   20g
- Fat   20g
- Fiber   4g
- Sugar   6g

NOTES:

Store in an airtight container in the fridge for up to 3 days. Reheat in a skillet before serving.

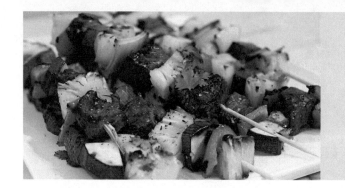

BEEF AND PINEAPPLE SKEWERS

INGREDIENTS

COOK TIME: 10   TOTAL TIME: 20
PREP TIME: 10   SERVINGS: 2

- 8 oz Beef (cubed)
- 1 cup Pineapple (cubed)
- 1 Bell pepper (cubed, for reintroduction)
- 1 Zucchini (sliced)
- 1 Onion (quartered)
- 2 tbsp Olive oil

- 1/2 tsp Sea salt
- 1/4 tsp Black pepper (optional)
- 1 tbsp Fresh cilantro (chopped)

DIRECTION

01   Preheat grill to medium-high heat.

02   Thread beef, pineapple, bell pepper, zucchini, and onion onto skewers.

03   Brush with olive oil, salt, and pepper (optional).

04   Grill for 10-15 minutes, turning occasionally.

05   Sprinkle with fresh cilantro and serve hot.

NUTRITIONAL INFO PER SERVING

- Calories   350
- Protein   30g
- Carbs   20g
- Fat   18g
- Fiber   4g
- Sugar   10g

NOTES:
Store leftovers in an airtight container in the fridge for up to 2 days. Reheat on the grill or in the oven before serving.

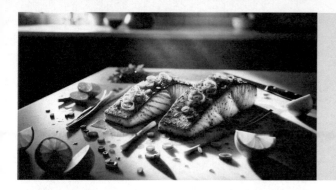

LEMON HERB MAHI MAHI WITH GARLIC AND GREEN ONIONS

INGREDIENTS

COOK TIME: 15
PREP TIME: 10
TOTAL TIME: 25
SERVINGS: 2

- 2 Mahi Mahi fillets
- 1 Lemon (juiced)
- 2 Garlic cloves (minced)
- 2 Green onions (chopped)
- 2 tbsp Olive oil
- 1/2 tsp Sea salt
- 1/4 tsp Black pepper (optional)
- 1 tbsp Fresh parsley (chopped)

DIRECTION

01 Preheat oven to 375°F (190°C).

02 Place Mahi Mahi fillets on a baking sheet.

03 Drizzle with olive oil, lemon juice, garlic, salt, and pepper (optional).

04 Sprinkle with green onions and parsley.

05 Bake for 15 minutes or until cooked through.

06 Serve hot.

NUTRITIONAL INFO PER SERVING

- Calories 250
- Protein 24g
- Carbs 5g
- Fat 16g
- Fiber 1g
- Sugar 1g

NOTES:

Store in an airtight container in the fridge for up to 2 days. Reheat in the oven before serving.

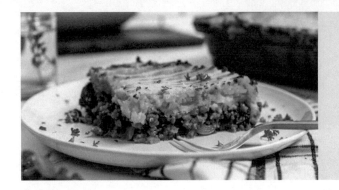

PORK AND SWEET POTATO SHEPHERD'S PIE

INGREDIENTS

COOK TIME: 30
PREP TIME: 15

TOTAL TIME: 45
SERVINGS: 2

- 8 oz Ground pork
- 2 Sweet potatoes (mashed)
- 1/2 Onion (diced)
- 2 cups Spinach (chopped)
- 1 Carrot (diced)
- 2 tbsp Olive oil
- 1/2 tsp Sea salt
- 1/4 tsp Black pepper (optional)
- 1/2 cup Bone broth

DIRECTION

01 Preheat oven to 375°F (190°C).

02 Heat olive oil in a skillet over medium heat.

03 Add onion and carrot, cook until tender.

04 Add ground pork, cook until browned.

05 Stir in spinach, bone broth, salt, and pepper (optional).

06 Transfer to a baking dish, top with mashed sweet potatoes, and bake for 20 minutes.

NUTRITIONAL INFO PER SERVING

- Calories 450
- Protein 28g
- Carbs 45g
- Fat 18g
- Fiber 7g
- Sugar 7g

NOTES:

Store in an airtight container in the fridge for up to 3 days. Reheat in the oven before serving.

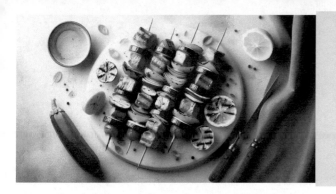

GRILLED BELL PEPPERS AND PORK SKEWERS
(FOR REINTRODUCTION)

INGREDIENTS

COOK TIME: 10
PREP TIME: 15
TOTAL TIME: 25
SERVINGS: 2

- 8 oz Pork (cubed)
- 2 Bell peppers (cubed)
- 1 Zucchini (sliced)
- 1 Onion (quartered)
- 1 Lemon (juiced)
- 2 tbsp Olive oil
- 1/2 tsp Sea salt
- 1/4 tsp Black pepper (optional)
- 1 tbsp Fresh rosemary (chopped)

DIRECTION

01 Preheat grill to medium-high heat.

02 In a bowl, mix lemon juice, olive oil, salt, pepper (optional), and rosemary.

03 Thread pork, bell peppers, zucchini, and onion onto skewers.

04 Brush with marinade.

05 Grill for 10-15 minutes, turning occasionally.

06 Serve hot.

NUTRITIONAL INFO PER SERVING

- Calories   300
- Protein   24g
- Carbs   20g
- Fat   18g
- Fiber   4g
- Sugar   5g

NOTES:
Store leftovers in an airtight container in the fridge for up to 2 days. Reheat on the grill or in the oven before serving.

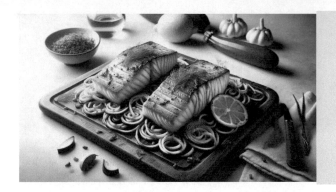

BAKED MAHI MAHI WITH FRESH DILL AND ZUCCHINI NOODLES

INGREDIENTS

COOK TIME: 15
PREP TIME: 10

TOTAL TIME: 25
SERVINGS: 2

- 2 Mahi Mahi fillets
- 1 Zucchini (spiralized)
- 2 tbsp Fresh dill (chopped)
- 1 Lemon (juiced)
- 2 Garlic cloves (minced)
- 2 tbsp Olive oil
- 1/2 tsp Sea salt
- 1/4 tsp Black pepper (optional)

DIRECTION

01 Preheat oven to 375°F (190°C).

02 Place Mahi Mahi fillets on a baking sheet.

03 Drizzle with olive oil, lemon juice, garlic, salt, pepper (optional), and dill.

04 Bake for 15 minutes or until cooked through.

05 Spiralize zucchini and serve raw or lightly sautéed.

06 Serve Mahi Mahi over zucchini noodles.

NUTRITIONAL INFO PER SERVING

- Calories   220
- Protein   24g
- Carbs   5g
- Fat   10g
- Fiber   1g
- Sugar   2g

NOTES:

Store in an airtight container in the fridge for up to 2 days. Reheat Mahi Mahi in the oven before serving. Zucchini noodles can be stored raw.

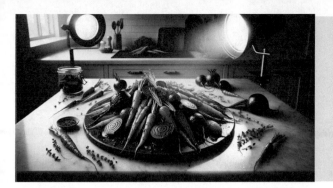

ROASTED BEETS AND CARROTS WITH FRESH THYME

INGREDIENTS

COOK TIME: 30
PREP TIME: 10
TOTAL TIME: 40
SERVINGS: 2

- 2 Beets (diced)
- 2 Carrots (diced)
- 2 tbsp Olive oil
- 1 tbsp Fresh thyme (chopped)
- 1/2 tsp Sea salt
- 1/4 tsp Black pepper (optional)

DIRECTION

01 Preheat oven to 400°F (200°C).

02 Toss beets and carrots with olive oil, thyme, salt, and pepper (optional).

03 Spread on a baking sheet.

04 Roast for 30 minutes or until tender, stirring halfway through.

05 Serve hot.

NUTRITIONAL INFO PER SERVING

- Calories 180
- Protein 2g
- Carbs 20g
- Fat 10g
- Fiber 6g
- Sugar 10g

NOTES:
Store in an airtight container in the fridge for up to 3 days. Reheat in the oven before serving.

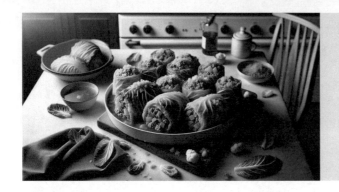

PORK STUFFED GREEN CABBAGE ROLLS

INGREDIENTS

COOK TIME: 30   TOTAL TIME: 45
PREP TIME: 15   SERVINGS: 2

- 8 Green cabbage leaves
- 8 oz Ground pork
- 1/2 Onion (diced)
- 1 Carrot (diced)
- 1 cup Cauliflower rice
- 2 tbsp Olive oil
- 1/2 tsp Sea salt
- 1/4 tsp Black pepper (optional)
- 1 cup Bone broth
- 1 tbsp Fresh parsley (chopped)

DIRECTION

01 Preheat oven to 375°F (190°C).

02 Blanch cabbage leaves in boiling water for 2 minutes.

03 Heat olive oil in a skillet over medium heat.

04 Add onion and carrot, cook until tender.

05 Add ground pork, cook until browned.

06 Mix in cauliflower rice, salt, pepper (optional), and parsley. Roll mixture into cabbage leaves and place in a baking dish. Pour bone broth over rolls and bake for 20 minutes.

NUTRITIONAL INFO PER SERVING

- Calories   350
- Protein   25g
- Carbs   20g
- Fat   16g
- Fiber   5g
- Sugar   4g

NOTES:

Store in an airtight container in the fridge for up to 2 days. Reheat in the oven before serving.

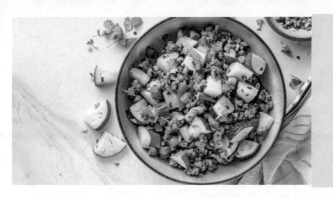

PINEAPPLE AND PORK STIR-FRY WITH FRESH CILANTRO

INGREDIENTS

COOK TIME: 10
PREP TIME: 10
TOTAL TIME: 20
SERVINGS: 2

- 8 oz Ground pork
- 1 cup Pineapple (diced)
- 1 Zucchini (sliced)
- 1 Bell pepper (sliced, for reintroduction)
- 2 Garlic cloves (minced)
- 2 tbsp Olive oil
- 1/4 cup Fresh cilantro (chopped)
- 1/2 tsp Sea salt
- 1/4 tsp Black pepper (optional)

DIRECTION

01 Heat olive oil in a skillet over medium heat.

02 Add garlic and cook until fragrant.

03 Add ground pork and cook until browned.

04 Add pineapple, zucchini, and bell pepper; cook until tender.

05 Stir in cilantro, salt, and pepper (optional).

06 Serve hot.

NUTRITIONAL INFO PER SERVING

- Calories   320
- Protein   24g
- Carbs   20g
- Fat   18g
- Fiber   4g
- Sugar   12g

NOTES:
Store in an airtight container in the fridge for up to 2 days. Reheat in a skillet before serving.

CHAPTER 08

SNACK RECIPES

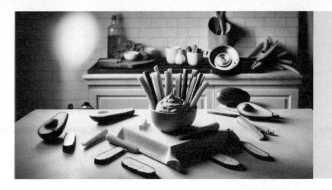

CARROT & CUCUMBER STICKS W/ AVOCADO DIP

INGREDIENTS

COOK TIME: 0
PREP TIME: 10
TOTAL TIME: 10
SERVINGS: 2

- 2 Carrots (sliced)
- 1 Cucumber (sliced)
- 1 Avocado
- 1 tbsp Lemon juice
- 1 tbsp Olive oil
- 1/2 tsp Salt
- 1/4 tsp Garlic powder

DIRECTION

01 Slice carrots and cucumber into sticks.

02 Mash avocado with lemon juice, olive oil, salt, and garlic powder until smooth.

03 Serve the dip with vegetable sticks.

NUTRITIONAL INFO PER SERVING

- Calories 250
- Protein 3g
- Carbs 24g
- Fat 18g
- Fiber 11g
- Sugar 6g

NOTES:

Best eaten immediately. Can be stored in an airtight container for up to a day.

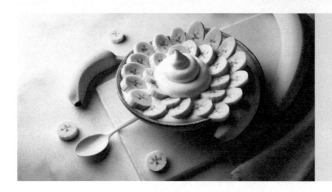

BANANA WITH COCONUT YOGURT

INGREDIENTS

COOK TIME: 0
PREP TIME: 5

TOTAL TIME: 5
SERVINGS: 2

- 1 Banana (sliced)
- 1 cup Coconut yogurt

DIRECTION

01 Slice the banana.

02 Serve banana slices with coconut yogurt.

NUTRITIONAL INFO PER SERVING

- Calories 200
- Protein 2g
- Carbs 28g
- Fat 10g
- Fiber 4g
- Sugar 15g

NOTES:

Best served immediately. Store any extra coconut yogurt in the fridge.

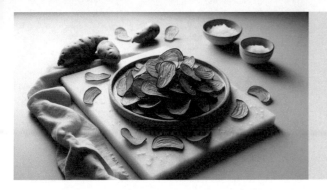

ROASTED SWEET POTATO CHIPS

INGREDIENTS

COOK TIME: 20
PREP TIME: 10
TOTAL TIME: 30
SERVINGS: 2

- 2 Sweet Potatoes (thinly sliced)
- 2 tbsp Olive oil
- 1/2 tsp Sea salt
- 1/4 tsp Garlic powder

DIRECTION

01   Preheat oven to 400°F (200°C).

02   Toss sweet potato slices with olive oil, salt, and garlic powder.

03   Spread slices on a baking sheet.

04   Bake for 20 minutes, flipping halfway through.

05   Let cool before serving.

NUTRITIONAL INFO PER SERVING

- Calories   160
- Protein   2g
- Carbs   30g
- Fat   5g
- Fiber   4g
- Sugar   7g

NOTES:
Store in an airtight container for up to 3 days. Reheat in the oven for a few minutes to crisp up.

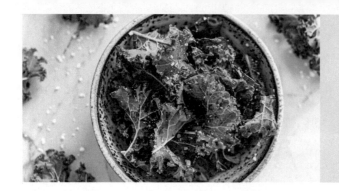

SAUTÉED KALE CHIPS WITH SEA SALT

INGREDIENTS

COOK TIME: 10
PREP TIME: 5

TOTAL TIME: 15
SERVINGS: 2

- 4 cups Kale (destemmed, chopped)
- 2 tbsp Olive oil
- 1/2 tsp Sea salt

DIRECTION

01 Heat olive oil in a skillet over medium heat.

02 Add kale and sauté until crispy, about 10 minutes.

03 Season with sea salt.

NUTRITIONAL INFO PER SERVING

- Calories 110
- Protein 2g
- Carbs 7g
- Fat 9g
- Fiber 2g
- Sugar 0g

NOTES:

Best eaten immediately. Can be stored in an airtight container for up to a day.

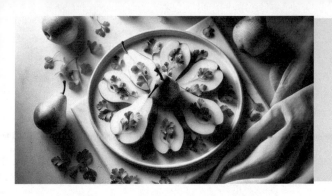

FRESH PEAR SLICES WITH FRESH CILANTRO

INGREDIENTS

COOK TIME: 0
PREP TIME: 5

TOTAL TIME: 5
SERVINGS: 2

- 2 Pears (sliced)

- 2 tbsp Fresh cilantro (chopped)

DIRECTION

01   Slice pears.

02   Sprinkle chopped cilantro over pear slices.

NUTRITIONAL INFO PER SERVING

- Calories   100
- Protein   1g
- Carbs   26g
- Fat   0g
- Fiber   6g
- Sugar   16g

NOTES:

Serve immediately. Store sliced pears in the fridge for up to a day.

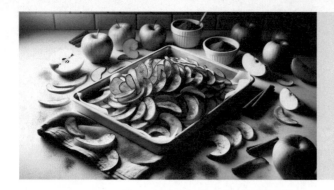

BAKED APPLE CHIPS WITH CINNAMON

INGREDIENTS

COOK TIME: 60
PREP TIME: 10
TOTAL TIME: 70
SERVINGS: 2

- 2 Apples (thinly sliced)
- 1 tsp Cinnamon

DIRECTION

01 Preheat oven to 200°F (90°C).

02 Arrange apple slices on a baking sheet.

03 Sprinkle with cinnamon.

04 Bake for 1 hour, flipping halfway through.

05 Let cool before serving.

NUTRITIONAL INFO PER SERVING

- Calories 90
- Protein 0g
- Carbs 25g
- Fat 0g
- Fiber 4g
- Sugar 19g

NOTES:
Store in an airtight container for up to a week.

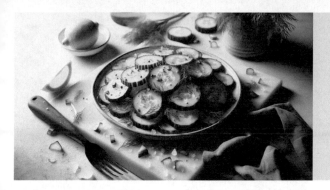

CUCUMBER SLICES WITH FRESH DILL

INGREDIENTS

COOK TIME: 0
PREP TIME: 5

TOTAL TIME: 5
SERVINGS: 2

- 1 Cucumber (sliced)
- 2 tbsp Fresh dill (chopped)
- 1 tbsp Lemon juice
- 1 tbsp Olive oil
- 1/2 tsp Sea salt

DIRECTION

01 Slice cucumber.

02 Toss with fresh dill, lemon juice, olive oil, and sea salt.

NUTRITIONAL INFO PER SERVING

- Calories 60
- Protein 0g
- Carbs 4g
- Fat 5g
- Fiber 1g
- Sugar 1g

NOTES:

Best served immediately. Store any leftovers in an airtight container in the fridge for up to 1 day.

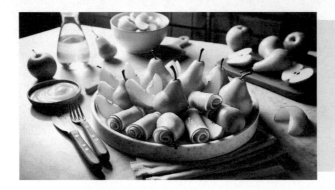

FRESH PEAR SLICES WITH TURKEY ROLL-UPS

INGREDIENTS

COOK TIME: 0
PREP TIME: 10

TOTAL TIME: 10
SERVINGS: 2

- 1 Pear (sliced)

- 4 oz Turkey (sliced)

DIRECTION

01   Slice pear.

02   Roll turkey slices and serve with pear slices.

NUTRITIONAL INFO PER SERVING

- Calories   120
- Protein   12g
- Carbs   18g
- Fat   2g
- Fiber   4g
- Sugar   12g

NOTES:

Best served immediately. Store leftover turkey in an airtight container in the fridge.

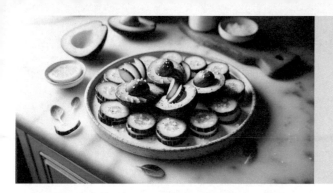

CUCUMBER AND AVOCADO BITES

INGREDIENTS

COOK TIME: 0
PREP TIME: 10
TOTAL TIME: 10
SERVINGS: 2

- 1 Cucumber (sliced)
- 1 Avocado (sliced)
- 1 Lemon (juiced)
- 1/4 tsp Sea salt

DIRECTION

01 Slice cucumber and avocado.

02 Squeeze lemon juice over avocado slices.

03 Sprinkle sea salt over avocado.

04 Place avocado slices on cucumber slices.

05 Serve immediately.

NUTRITIONAL INFO PER SERVING

- Calories   180
- Protein   2g
- Carbs   20g
- Fat   14g
- Fiber   10g
- Sugar   1g

NOTES:

Best served immediately. Store leftover avocado with lemon juice to prevent browning.

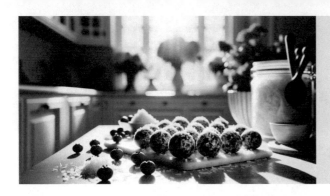

BLUEBERRY AND COCONUT ENERGY BALLS

INGREDIENTS

COOK TIME: 0
PREP TIME: 15

TOTAL TIME: 15
SERVINGS: 2

- 1 cup Blueberries
- 1 cup Shredded coconut
- 2 tbsp Honey
- 1/2 cup Coconut flour
- 1/2 tsp Vanilla extract (AIP compliant)

DIRECTION

01 Blend blueberries until smooth.

02 In a bowl, mix blueberry puree, shredded coconut, honey, coconut flour, and vanilla extract.

03 Form mixture into balls.

04 Chill in the fridge for 30 minutes before serving.

NUTRITIONAL INFO PER SERVING

- Calories 150
- Protein   2g
- Carbs   20g
- Fat   8g
- Fiber   6g
- Sugar   14g

NOTES:
Store in an airtight container in the fridge for up to 3 days.

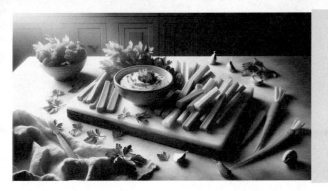

CARROT AND CELERY STICKS WITH FRESH PARSLEY DIP

INGREDIENTS

COOK TIME: 0
PREP TIME: 10
TOTAL TIME: 10
SERVINGS: 2

- 2 Carrots (sliced)
- 2 Celery stalks (sliced)
- 1/2 cup Coconut yogurt
- 2 tbsp Fresh parsley (chopped)
- 1 Garlic clove (minced)
- 1 tbsp Lemon juice
- 1/4 tsp Sea salt

DIRECTION

01 Slice carrots and celery.

02 In a bowl, mix coconut yogurt, parsley, garlic, lemon juice, and sea salt.

03 Serve vegetable sticks with dip.

NUTRITIONAL INFO PER SERVING

- Calories   100
- Protein   1g
- Carbs   18g
- Fat   4g
- Fiber   4g
- Sugar   6g

NOTES:
Store dip in an airtight container in the fridge for up to 2 days.

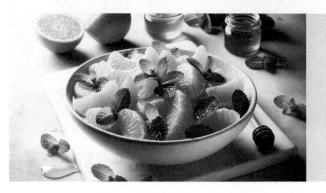

ORANGE AND FRESH MINT FRUIT SALAD

INGREDIENTS

COOK TIME: 0
PREP TIME: 10
TOTAL TIME: 10
SERVINGS: 2

- 2 Oranges (peeled, segmented)
- 2 tbsp Fresh mint (chopped)
- 1 tbsp Honey

DIRECTION

01   Peel and segment oranges.

02   Toss orange segments with fresh mint and honey.

03   Serve immediately.

NUTRITIONAL INFO PER SERVING

- Calories   120
- Protein   1g
- Carbs   30g
- Fat   0g
- Fiber   4g
- Sugar   24g

NOTES:

Best served immediately. Store in an airtight container in the fridge for up to 1 day.

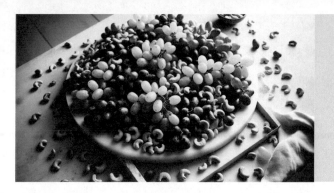

FRESH GRAPES AND CASHEWS

(FOR REINTRODUCTION)

INGREDIENTS

COOK TIME: 0
PREP TIME: 5

TOTAL TIME: 5
SERVINGS: 2

- 1 cup Grapes (halved)
- 1/4 cup Cashews (raw)

DIRECTION

01 Halve the grapes.

02 Serve grapes with cashews.

NUTRITIONAL INFO PER SERVING

- Calories 200
- Protein 5g
- Carbs 26g
- Fat 10g
- Fiber 2g
- Sugar 22g

NOTES:

Best served immediately. Store leftover grapes in an airtight container in the fridge.

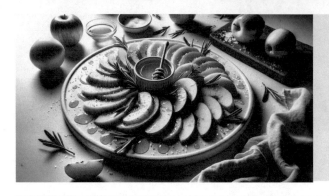

APPLE SLICES WITH FRESH ROSEMARY AND LEMON DRIZZLE

INGREDIENTS

COOK TIME: 0
PREP TIME: 10

TOTAL TIME: 10
SERVINGS: 2

- 2 Apples (sliced)
- 1 Lemon (juiced)
- 1 tbsp Fresh rosemary (chopped)
- 1 tbsp Honey
- 1/4 tsp Sea salt

DIRECTION

01   Slice apples.

02   In a small bowl, mix lemon juice, rosemary, honey, and sea salt.

03   Drizzle over apple slices.

04   Serve immediately.

NUTRITIONAL INFO PER SERVING

- Calories   150
- Protein   1g
- Carbs   40g
- Fat   0g
- Fiber   6g
- Sugar   30g

NOTES:

Best served immediately. Store leftover apple slices with lemon juice to prevent browning.

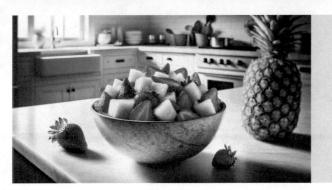

PINEAPPLE AND STRAWBERRY FRUIT SALAD

INGREDIENTS

COOK TIME: 0
PREP TIME: 10

TOTAL TIME: 10
SERVINGS: 2

- 1 cup Pineapple (diced)
- 1 cup Strawberries (sliced)

DIRECTION

01   Dice pineapple.

02   Slice strawberries.

03   Combine in a bowl and mix gently.

04   Serve immediately.

NUTRITIONAL INFO PER SERVING

- Calories   100
- Protein   1g
- Carbs   25g
- Fat   0g
- Fiber   4g
- Sugar   18g

NOTES:

Store in an airtight container in the fridge for up to 3 days.

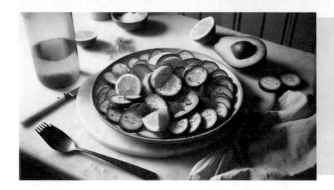

CUCUMBER AND AVOCADO SLICES WITH FRESH DILL

INGREDIENTS

COOK TIME: 0
PREP TIME: 10
TOTAL TIME: 10
SERVINGS: 2

- 1 Cucumber (sliced)
- 1 Avocado (sliced)
- 1 tbsp Lemon juice
- 1 tbsp Fresh dill (chopped)
- 1/4 tsp Sea salt

DIRECTION

01   Slice cucumber and avocado.

02   Drizzle avocado slices with lemon juice.

03   Sprinkle fresh dill and sea salt over avocado.

04   Serve cucumber and avocado slices together.

NUTRITIONAL INFO PER SERVING

- Calories   160
- Protein   2g
- Carbs   12g
- Fat   12g
- Fiber   8g
- Sugar   1g

NOTES:

Best served immediately. Store avocado with lemon juice to prevent browning.

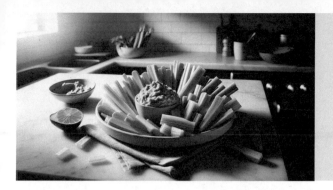

CARROT AND CELERY STICKS WITH GUACAMOLE

INGREDIENTS

COOK TIME: 0
PREP TIME: 10

TOTAL TIME: 10
SERVINGS: 2

- 2 Carrots (sliced)
- 2 Celery stalks (sliced)
- 2 Avocados
- 1 Lime (juiced)
- 1/4 cup Onion (diced)
- 1 Garlic clove (minced)
- 1/4 tsp Sea salt
- 1/4 tsp Black pepper (optional)

DIRECTION

01 Slice carrots and celery.

02 Mash avocados with lime juice, onion, garlic, salt, and pepper (optional) to make guacamole.

NUTRITIONAL INFO PER SERVING

- Calories 220
- Protein 3g
- Carbs 20g
- Fat 16g
- Fiber 12g
- Sugar 6g

03 Serve vegetable sticks with guacamole.

NOTES:

Store guacamole in an airtight container in the fridge for up to 1 day.

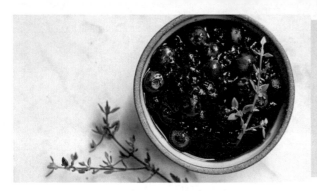

BLUEBERRIES AND FRESH THYME COMPOTE

INGREDIENTS

COOK TIME: 10
PREP TIME: 5
TOTAL TIME: 15
SERVINGS: 2

- 1 cup Blueberries
- 1 tbsp Fresh thyme (chopped)
- 1 tbsp Honey
- 1/4 cup Water

DIRECTION

01 Combine blueberries, thyme, honey, and water in a saucepan.

02 Cook over medium heat until blueberries burst and mixture thickens.

03 Let cool before serving.

NUTRITIONAL INFO PER SERVING

- Calories   80
- Protein   1g
- Carbs   20g
- Fat   0g
- Fiber   2g
- Sugar   16g

NOTES:
Store in an airtight container in the fridge for up to 3 days.

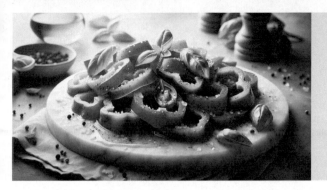

BELL PEPPER SLICES WITH FRESH BASIL

(REINTRODUCTION: BELL PEPPERS)

INGREDIENTS

COOK TIME: 0
PREP TIME: 10
TOTAL TIME: 10
SERVINGS: 2

- 2 Bell peppers (sliced)

- 2 tbsp Fresh basil (chopped)

- 1 tbsp Olive oil

- 1/4 tsp Sea salt

DIRECTION

01   Slice bell peppers.

02   Toss with olive oil and sea salt.

03   Sprinkle fresh basil over the top.

04   Serve immediately.

NUTRITIONAL INFO PER SERVING

- Calories   120
- Protein   2g
- Carbs   14g
- Fat   9g
- Fiber   4g
- Sugar   8g

NOTES:

Best served immediately. Store in an airtight container in the fridge for up to 1 day.

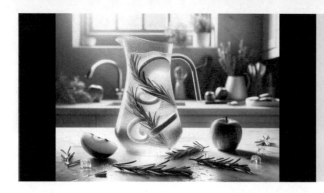

APPLE AND FRESH ROSEMARY INFUSED WATER

INGREDIENTS

COOK TIME: 0
PREP TIME: 5
TOTAL TIME: 5
SERVINGS: 2

- 1 Apple (sliced)

- 1 tbsp Fresh rosemary (chopped)

- 4 cups Water

DIRECTION

01   Slice apple.

02   Combine apple slices, rosemary, and water in a pitcher.

NUTRITIONAL INFO PER SERVING

- Calories   10
- Protein   0g
- Carbs   3g
- Fat   0g
- Fiber   1g
- Sugar   2g

03   Let infuse in the fridge for at least 1 hour before serving.

NOTES:
Store infused water in the fridge for up to 1 day.

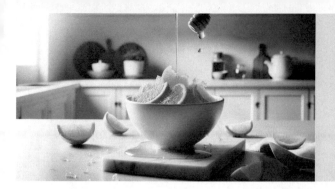

ORANGE AND LEMON ZEST FRUIT CUPS

INGREDIENTS

COOK TIME: 0
PREP TIME: 10

TOTAL TIME: 10
SERVINGS: 2

- 2 Oranges (segmented)

- 1 Lemon (zested)

- 1 tbsp Honey

DIRECTION

01 Segment oranges.

02 Combine orange segments, lemon zest, and honey in a bowl.

03 Toss gently to combine.

04 Serve immediately.

NUTRITIONAL INFO PER SERVING

- Calories   120
- Protein   1g
- Carbs   30g
- Fat   0g
- Fiber   5g
- Sugar   24g

NOTES:

Best served immediately. Store leftovers in an airtight container in the fridge for up to 1 day.

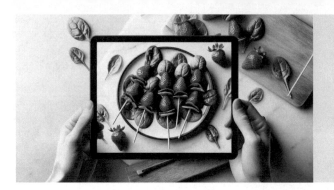

STRAWBERRY AND SPINACH MINI SKEWERS

INGREDIENTS

COOK TIME: 0
PREP TIME: 10

TOTAL TIME: 10
SERVINGS: 2

- 1 cup Strawberries (halved)

- 1 cup Spinach leaves

DIRECTION

01 Thread strawberries and spinach leaves onto mini skewers.

02 Serve immediately.

NUTRITIONAL INFO PER SERVING

- Calories   50
- Protein   1g
- Carbs   12g
- Fat   0g
- Fiber   2g
- Sugar   8g

NOTES:

Best served immediately. Store leftovers in an airtight container in the fridge for up to 1 day.

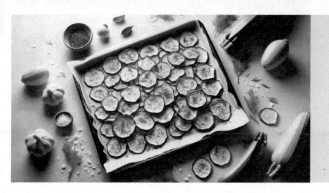

ZUCCHINI CHIPS WITH FRESH DILL

INGREDIENTS

COOK TIME: 90
PREP TIME: 10
TOTAL TIME: 100
SERVINGS: 2

- 2 Zucchini (sliced thin)
- 2 tbsp Olive oil
- 1 tbsp Fresh dill (chopped)
- 1/2 tsp Sea salt
- 1/4 tsp Garlic powder

DIRECTION

01   Preheat oven to 225°F (110°C).

02   Toss zucchini slices with olive oil, dill, sea salt, and garlic powder.

03   Arrange in a single layer on a baking sheet.

04   Bake for 90 minutes or until crispy.

05   Let cool before serving.

NUTRITIONAL INFO PER SERVING

- Calories   100
- Protein   2g
- Carbs   8g
- Fat   7g
- Fiber   2g
- Sugar   3g

NOTES:
Store in an airtight container for up to 2 days.

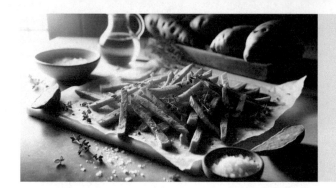

SWEET POTATO FRIES WITH FRESH THYME

INGREDIENTS

COOK TIME: 30
PREP TIME: 10

TOTAL TIME: 40
SERVINGS: 2

- 2 Sweet potatoes (sliced into fries)
- 2 tbsp Olive oil
- 1 tbsp Fresh thyme (chopped)
- 1/2 tsp Sea salt
- 1/4 tsp Black pepper (optional)

DIRECTION

01 Preheat oven to 425°F (220°C).

02 Toss sweet potato fries with olive oil, thyme, sea salt, and pepper (optional).

03 Arrange on a baking sheet.

04 Bake for 30 minutes or until crispy, flipping halfway through.

05 Serve hot.

NUTRITIONAL INFO PER SERVING

- Calories 200
- Protein 2g
- Carbs 35g
- Fat 8g
- Fiber 5g
- Sugar 7g

NOTES:

Store in an airtight container in the fridge for up to 2 days. Reheat in the oven before serving.

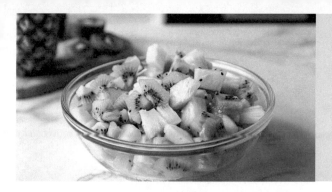

PINEAPPLE AND KIWI FRUIT SALAD
(FOR REINTRODUCTION)

INGREDIENTS

COOK TIME: 0
PREP TIME: 10
TOTAL TIME: 10
SERVINGS: 2

- 1 cup Pineapple (diced)

- 2 Kiwi (peeled, diced)

DIRECTION

01   Dice pineapple and kiwi.

02   Combine in a bowl and mix gently.

03   Serve immediately.

NUTRITIONAL INFO PER SERVING

- Calories   100
- Protein   1g
- Carbs   26g
- Fat   0g
- Fiber   3g
- Sugar   18g

NOTES:

Best served immediately. Store leftovers in an airtight container in the fridge for up to 1 day.

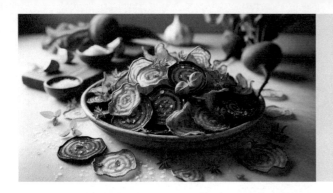

BEET CHIPS WITH FRESH OREGANO

INGREDIENTS

COOK TIME: 45
PREP TIME: 10

TOTAL TIME: 55
SERVINGS: 2

- 2 Beets (sliced thin)
- 2 tbsp Olive oil
- 1 tbsp Fresh oregano (chopped)
- 1/2 tsp Sea salt
- 1/4 tsp Garlic powder

DIRECTION

01　Preheat oven to 375°F (190°C).

02　Toss beet slices with olive oil, oregano, sea salt, and garlic powder.

03　Arrange in a single layer on a baking sheet.

04　Bake for 45 minutes or until crispy, flipping halfway through.

05　Let cool before serving.

NUTRITIONAL INFO PER SERVING

- Calories　150
- Protein　2g
- Carbs　20g
- Fat　8g
- Fiber　4g
- Sugar　10g

NOTES:
Store in an airtight container for up to 2 days.

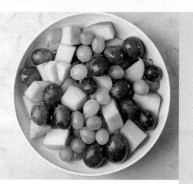

MANGO AND GRAPES FRUIT SALAD
(FOR REINTRODUCTION)

INGREDIENTS

COOK TIME: 0
PREP TIME: 10

TOTAL TIME: 10
SERVINGS: 2

- 1 Mango (diced)

- 1 cup Grapes (halved)

DIRECTION

01 Dice mango and halve grapes.

02 Combine in a bowl and mix gently.

03 Serve immediately.

NUTRITIONAL INFO PER SERVING

- Calories 120
- Protein 1g
- Carbs 31g
- Fat 0g
- Fiber 3g
- Sugar 27g

NOTES:

Best served immediately. Store leftovers in an airtight container in the fridge for up to 1 day.

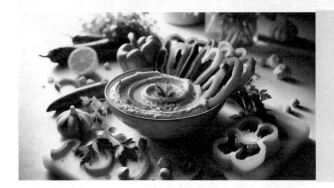

BELL PEPPER AND FRESH PARSLEY HUMMUS DIP

(WITH CHICKPEAS - REINTRODUCTION)

INGREDIENTS

COOK TIME: 0
PREP TIME: 10

TOTAL TIME: 10
SERVINGS: 2

- 1 Bell pepper (sliced)
- 1 cup Chickpeas
- 1/4 cup Olive oil
- 1 Garlic clove

- 1 tbsp Fresh parsley (chopped)
- 1/4 tsp Cumin (optional)
- 1/4 tsp Sea salt
- 1 tbsp Lemon juice

DIRECTION

01 In a blender, combine chickpeas, olive oil, garlic, lemon juice, sea salt, and cumin (optional).

02 Blend until smooth.

03 Transfer to a bowl and sprinkle with fresh parsley.

04 Serve with bell pepper slices.

NUTRITIONAL INFO PER SERVING

- Calories 250
- Protein 6g
- Carbs 22g
- Fat 14g
- Fiber 6g
- Sugar 2g

NOTES:
Store hummus in an airtight container in the fridge for up to 3 days.

THANK YOU

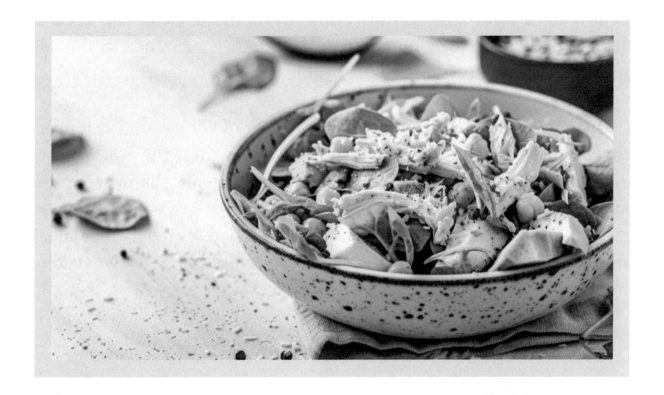

To quote Hippocrates, 'Let food be thy medicine and medicine be thy food.' This adage holds especially true for those of us following the Autoimmune Protocol (AIP) diet. Through the careful selection of nutrient-dense, anti-inflammatory foods, we aim to heal our bodies from within, addressing the root causes of autoimmune conditions rather than merely managing symptoms. The recipes in this book are more than just meals; they are steps towards reclaiming your health and vitality.

As you continue your AIP journey, the process of reintroducing foods becomes crucial. This stage allows you to identify specific triggers and customize your diet to suit your unique needs. It's important to approach reintroduction with patience and mindfulness, taking note of how each food affects your body. By doing so, you can create a sustainable eating plan that not only supports your health but also brings joy and variety back to your table.

Thank you for allowing this book to be a part of your wellness journey. Your commitment to exploring and embracing the AIP diet is commendable, and I hope these recipes have made the process both enjoyable and enlightening. Remember, every step you take towards better health is a victory. Here's to a future filled with delicious meals, improved well-being, and a deeper understanding of what truly nourishes you.

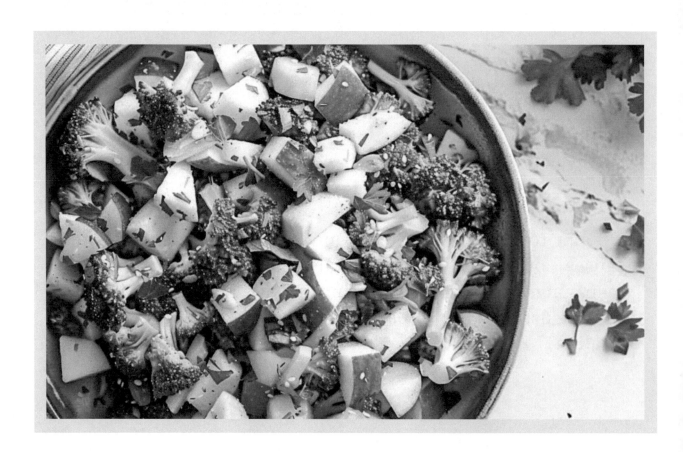

As an independent publisher your thoughts mean the world to me. Please consider leaving an honest review of this cookbook so I can know what you found useful and how I can improve to make this a valuable addition to your healthy living journey. Scan the QR code below to go straight to the review page!

Kevin Wagonfoot

Made in United States
Troutdale, OR
11/02/2024

24378095R00082